To John

With my best wishes to you for a long and healthy life.

Celebrate each day!
Celebrate life!!
Celebrate your wrinkles!!!

[signature]

A New Wrinkle

What I Learned from Older People Who Never Acted Their Age

Dr. Eric Z. Shapira, DDS, MA, MHA

iUniverse, Inc.
New York   Bloomington

A New Wrinkle
What I Learned from Older People Who Never Acted Their Age

Copyright © 2009 by Dr. Eric Z. Shapira, DDS, MA, MHA

All rights reserved. No part of this book may be used or reproduced by any means, graphic, electronic, or mechanical, including photocopying, recording, taping or by any information storage retrieval system without the written permission of the publisher except in the case of brief quotations embodied in critical articles and reviews.

The views expressed in this work are solely those of the author and do not necessarily reflect the views of the publisher, and the publisher hereby disclaims any responsibility for them.

iUniverse books may be ordered through booksellers or by contacting:

iUniverse
1663 Liberty Drive
Bloomington, IN 47403
www.iuniverse.com
1-800-Authors (1-800-288-4677)

Because of the dynamic nature of the Internet, any Web addresses or links contained in this book may have changed since publication and may no longer be valid.

ISBN: 978-1-4401-6396-8 (sc)
ISBN: 978-1-4401-6650-1 (dj)
ISBN: 978-1-4401-6649-5 (ebk)

Printed in the United States of America
iUniverse rev. date: 9/2/2009

("A Visit From Wisdom" from A TEAR AND A SMILE by Kahlil Gibran, translated by H.N. Nahmud, translation copyright 1950 by the Estate of Kahlil Gibran. Used by permission of Alfred A. Knopf, a division of Random House, Inc.)

(From TAO TE CHING by Lao Tsu, translated by Gia-fu Feng & Jane English, translation copyright © 1972 by Gia-fu Feng and Jane English, copyright renewed 2000 by Carol Wilson and Jane English. Used by permission of Alfred A. Knopf, a division of Random house, Inc.)

(PABLO NERUDA. "El tiempo que no se perdió.", from the work EL CORAZÓN AMARILLO © Fundación Pablo Neruda, 2009.)

(From THE ROAD AHEAD, REVISED EDITION by Bill Gates, copyright © 1995, 1996 by William Gates III. Used by permission of Viking Penguin, a division of Penguin Group (USA) Inc).

(From Hua Hu Ching: The Later Teachings of Lao Tzu, by Lao Tzu, translated and elucidated by Hua-Ching Ni, © 1979, 1995 by Hua-Ching Ni. Reprinted by arrangement with Shambhala Publications Inc., Boston, MA. www.shambhala.com.)

(From The Upanishads, translated by Eknath Easwaran, founder of the Blue Mountain Center of Meditation, copyright 1987, 2007; reprinted by permission of Nilgiri Press, P.O. Box 256, Tomales, CA 94971, www.easwaran.org.)

(From Bob Dylan, Dignity Copyright © 1991 Special Rider music. All rights reserved. International copyright secured. Reprinted by permission)

Contents

Acknowledgments vii
Preface ix
Chapter 1   Who Art Thou Romeo? 1
   Identity 1
   My Plight 4
   Aging with Identity 11
   Bubbie 17
   Nani 19
   Pep 25
   Leah and Joe 26
   Fanny and Saul 28
   Saul 31
Chapter 2   When the Music Changes, So Does the Dance 35
   Making Changes 35
   Can Age Make Us Change? 43
Chapter 3   Who's on First? 50
   Memory 50
   Behind Closed Doors 55
   Now That You've Got It, What Do You Do with It? 59
   What about the Caregiver? 68
   What to Look for in a Caregiver 71
   Memory Loss with Aging: What's Normal, What's Not 73
   Causes of Memory Loss 75
Chapter 4   An Apple a Day 79
   Aging and Chronic Disease 79
   If You Can Imagine It, You Can Do It 83
   Dementia and Alzheimer's Disease 88
   Mild Cognitive Impairment 90
   Early Warning Signs 91
   Chronic Disease and Aging 92
   How Can I Help My Memory? 102
Chapter 5   Early to Bed, Early to Rise 105
   Healthy Aging 105
   Meditation 112
   Alternative Treatment 114
   Acupuncture 115

Chiropractic Care	116
Exercise and Diet	120
Chapter 6 Sex Is Not the Answer. Sex Is the Question. "Yes" Is the Answer	130
Intimacy	130
Having Sex and Being Prepared	133
The Love Connection and the Internet	136
Caregivers and Intimacy	142
Intimacy	143
True Love or Scam	150
How to Have a Good Relationship	156
Chapter 7 To Be or Not To Be—Families in Crisis	162
Families in Transition	167
Family Dynamics	171
SWOT Analysis	174
Transitioning the Transition	176
Chapter 8 Now I Lay Me Down to Sleep	180
Death and Dying	180
The Grieving Process	188
Preparation and the Legacy	191
Extremely Important Documents	193
Special Awareness	197
Hospice Care	202
Chapter 9 Aging in Place	209
When You Don't Feel Like Moving Anymore!	209
Human Nature Takes Its Course	216
The Butterfly	220
Chapter 10 The Sequel	223
Have Dignity, Will Find Happiness	223
Discovering Dignity	226
Maintaining Happiness	234
Chapter 11 The End Is Only the Beginning and Then Some	243
Knowing Who We Are	246
A Short Story	248
Epilogue	253
Glossary of Terms	257
Related Reading	275
Helpful Resources	279
Index	289

Acknowledgments

I dedicate my book to my family: my father, Irving, who never made it to old age, but whose wisdom always told me to "study the situation" before I entered into any negotiation, big or small; my mother, Betty, who showed me through her humanitarian actions how to be a good and useful person; my baby sister, Jill, who I love with a passion and who will, I trust, be there when it is my turn to leave this earthly place, holding my hand and easing me through the passage; Gaylord, my brother-in-law, who has shown me patience working with those less fortunate; my younger brother, Harvey, and his wife, Carol who have always encouraged me and have been there to listen without passing judgment; my wife, Susan, who has given me love, support and encouragement and has taught me the power of play and the joys of spontaneity; my son, Zane, who, without knowing it, helped me find the child in me again and gave me a reason to live and enjoy life; my son's wife, Marlene, who gave me my first grandson, Griffin, and more to come with Verity, a new granddaughter; and Griffin, who brings me hope for a future world filled with respect for elders, creativity, wisdom, peace, good leadership, and contentment.

I also want to acknowledge my friends, especially Marilyn LeGette and Joan Solana, for their ability to listen and encourage me to continue writing this book, even though by everyone's standards, I haven't yet reached an age old enough to be telling people "how to." I would like to thank my editors, Nancy Margulies and Kate Mayer, for their understanding, their contributions, their time, their knowledge and their ability to encourage me. I would especially like to thank Nancy for her creativity and help with my illustrations as well. A BIG thank you to Noreen Cooper Heavlin, MLIS, (www.sortingthingsout.com) for her diligence, guidance, and wisdom in procuring copyright permission for me from the publishers and authors of innumerable quotes used in the body of my text. This book would not have been possible without her significant contribution.

Lastly, to those of you who ventured upon reading this book, I wish to thank you for your interest and foresight as well as for passing this title along to others who may benefit by reading *A New Wrinkle*.

We all have the ability to make choices about our lives that will make a difference in how we live our days. It is my hope that this book will help you make those choices for a life that is worth living. Enjoy the journey; the destination comes all too quickly in the scheme of things. **A portion of the profits from the sale of this book will go toward Rotary International's Humanitarian and Educational Foundation.**

Eric Z. Shapira, DDS, MA, MHA
Clinical Gerontologist, Educator, Retired Dentist
www.agingmentorservices.com
Written in Montara, California

Preface

My grandfather, perhaps quoting the famous second-century rabbinical teacher, Rabbi Akiva, once told me that, as we have two ears and one mouth, we should listen twice as much as we speak. By listening to older clients, I have discovered ways of living that add joy to one's years.

As a clinical gerontologist, I've spent many years lecturing, teaching, and helping individuals and families handle situations that emerge as loved ones age. I have written over a hundred articles and papers in professional journals and I lecture extensively in this country as well as abroad—I recently returned from China where I taught over five hundred medical professionals about hospice care and the challenges of aging. When giving talks, I'm often asked if I have written a book on aging. After looking over what's available, I realized that my unique perspective would be useful to many potential readers.

A New Wrinkle: What I Learned from Older People Who Never Acted Their Age, provides inspiring anecdotes as well as tips and insight into the complex issues facing a huge segment of our population. This book includes new material on managing families in crisis, handling transitions, and creating win-win situations for families and caregivers. Here you will find tips on how to choose caregivers and how to maintain a loving relationship if you are the caregiver of a spouse whose health is compromised.

There are eighty million baby boomers facing issues of aging while also caring for elderly parents. The audience for this book includes boomers who will soon enough become elders themselves and their parents who may be transitioning and reinventing themselves. I counsel a lot of people who are navigating complicated family dynamics. Often people just don't know what to do. Even our elders are wondering who they are and how they will continue to live a happy and productive life with dignity and good health in our throw-away society.

I can see now the rising waters of aging that are flooding the valleys of youth; however, if one is prepared for the flood and there are enough sandbags in place to keep things from getting ruined, the levees will hold back the torrent, and then one should be able to ride out the storm in comfort.

I always liked the Boy Scout motto "Be Prepared," and I wrote this book as a model of how to be prepared for the aging process.

Aging is a mystery for most of us, something that just happens—a complex labyrinth not too many of us ever pay attention to with respect to the signs and symptoms until we try to navigate our way out of it. There are too many variables that come into play when one really thinks about the scope of aging and how to cope. In light of the facts that we are living longer and that within a few years our society will be dominated by the more than 25 percent of the population over the age of sixty-five, we'd better put our glasses on and stop being myopic about this process.

Each of us has our own style of handling our unmet needs. Each of us has our own bank of emotions and reactions to change, whether it is a crisis or a celebration. Why not learn about yourself, how you think, how you feel in light of getting older, so that when you wake up in the midst of this process, you will realize that it is not a dream but a reality, inviting you to make the most of it.

That is what this book will help you do as you read along. I think it is important to stay flexible with respect to change, learning to go with the flow yet staying conscious about how fast the water is moving.

Chapter 1

Who Art Thou Romeo?

IDENTITY

"Who are you?" said the Caterpillar. Alice replied, rather shyly, "I—I hardly know, Sir, Just at present—at least I know who I was when I got up this morning, but I think I must have been changed several times since then."

—Lewis Carroll, *Alice's Adventures in Wonderland*

I was going along fine in my life. I had a profession, a family, friends, and many interests. However, for several years, I had been coping with pain from injuries to my neck, and the pain was escalating. It was forcing me to change the way I practiced dentistry and to seek alternative methods of pain control, because I did not want to take drugs. I had several epidural injections in the spine over a five-year period, only to get to a place where they did not work any more, and my pain was to the point I was not sure I could tolerate any more.

And then one day, as I was operating in my clinic, my left arm went dead. Yes, it was completely dead; no feeling and no movement. I could not pick up the instrument I was reaching for to finish the operation. Was I scared? Yes. Confused? Only for a moment while I thought about what happened. I got up and excused myself and then ran back into my private office and slammed my arm and hand against the wall several times. I waited, and then, finally, the feeling came back enough for me to finish the operation.

I immediately saw a neurosurgeon. He told me that if I had a car accident, a fall, or a slap to my face, I might not be able to walk ever again. He told me that I really did not have a choice and needed an operation as soon as possible. Where do I sign?

Needless to say, I had the surgery to fuse my cervical vertebrae, five through seven, and several cadaver bone grafts to boot. I thought I could go back to practicing, but I was fooling myself. The damage was done, and my movement was limited and my pain was lessened but still there. It took about three years to recover from that surgery, and in that time I went through many changes, both mental and physical. I went through much loss—creating grieving and depression, sadness and despair.

I lost my profession of over thirty years in the blink of an eye. So now what? Interesting to note, I looked into the mirror one day, and when I stared at myself, I was no longer a dentist. *Who am I?*, I thought? For all these years I related to myself as a dentist, and now that I was no longer going to be practicing dentistry I had to come to the realization that this was not me. Yes, I was a dentist, as far as my profession was concerned, but looking at the face in the mirror caused an epiphany. I realized that I was the same me, Eric Shapira, a person. I had come to realize, with the help of counseling, that I tended to relate myself to what I did and not to who I was. I think most of us tend to do this. This revelation helped me to recover my senses and eased the grief I felt at the time.

I had counseling from a very kind and understanding person. I spent a lot of time thinking about what would I do with my life and how would I accomplish new goals. I walked a lot to think and to heal. I talked with friends, and I went back to school to learn more about gerontology, earning a master's degree in clinical gerontology and a second master's degree in health administration. It required several years of persistent work, diligence, commitment, and tenacity. It took much soul searching as well as making a plan, setting goals, and having a vision.

All the things I write about in this book came to life for me. The traumatic event of my hand freezing during an operation caused a family crisis for me. The crisis involved financial loss for me and for my wife as well, as she had worked in my office as the manager for over twenty-five years. She lost her job too. There were bills to pay. There were continued medical treatment and rehabilitation, counseling for the depression and grieving that I was experiencing and the long, hard road of trying to decide what I wanted to do when I grew up. As it turned out, I had to have a second neck surgery about four years after the first one due to failing bone grafts, more bone loss, and a risk of breaking my neck. Not fun! I don't wish this on anyone.

I had to learn to love myself again. I had to make peace with my body and to accept the disability and the lack of movement and continued pain. I learned to push myself to heal and to learn new things like painting and writing that brought me pleasure. We all have our stories and we all have our own vicissitudes in life that impede our abilities to do things or make progress. But don't ever give up! I didn't. I stayed with my desire to help others by moving from one caregiver profession to another.

I wish to spread love and understanding and to teach others the power of the mind, the power of love, and the power of positive thinking. My most important goal is to encourage others to recapture their inner child and learn how to nurture it.

My Plight

Somehow in life I missed the section of the training manual that told me getting older was something that happens when you least expect it. This is a subtle experience for some, and yet, for others aging is much more of a shock. One day, I looked in the mirror, and there I was: looking at a stranger—a balding, graying, crow's foot, bags under formerly youthful eyes kind of guy. I had to laugh out loud because I kept visualizing my father! My laugh was but an oral reverberation of an internal scream. I knew down deep that I was looking at myself. What a revelation! Maybe some of you reading this can relate in some way, or maybe it just hit you and now you can laugh out loud along with me.

I had spent five years in graduate school studying to be a clinical gerontologist, after practicing dentistry for over thirty years, and suddenly I was my own client! Every time someone asked me why I went into gerontology I answered, "Because I wanted to know what I had to look forward to."

Well, so be it. There it was, staring me in the face with all its glory—me, an older me. I think it was a more patient me. Yes, maybe an even more accepting me.

No one tells us what to expect as we age. No one tells us how life wears on one's ability to maintain beauty and fine looks, strong abs or a sharp mind. In essence, *A New Wrinkle* means following a new line of experience or smiling a new smile about something you discover about yourself that may have been submerged all your life. Possibly the discovery was gleaned from other's experience, and then, in the middle of something, there it is, a mind burp that says "Ah ha!" For me it was "I'm gettin' up there!"

How do we define aging? How do we adapt to it? How can we make it our friend? Can we make it go away? And, how do we make peace with this time in our lives? Asking these questions and more are daily mantras for many of us. Some people just go about their business, never bothering to think about getting older until something happens that jolts them into an inability to think about anything else: a death of a close family member or friend of similar age; an operation that takes longer than expected to recover from; a gray hair or two discovered after a shower; sagging skin; flaccid muscles; a "new wrinkle"; a magazine with a youthful model that makes you think about self and the way you used to be; and maybe, trouble remembering where the car keys are a little too often.

Some of this is normal run-of-the mill aging, but some of this is abnormal in a sense. Much like the big C, cancer, the big A, aging, is scary. Most of us think we are invincible—right? We can leap tall buildings in a single bound. We can still make love all night long, wrestle with our kids and win, or water ski without falling. But when the day comes that you get pinned wrestling with your kid, thoughts of having sex are not exciting or you are not even motivated to perform any sex act, you fall off the skis one too many times, or you need a stepladder to leap those buildings, the aging (some call it the Big A) has arrived in all its glory.

How do we embrace this transition with love and acceptance to make the change one of grace and dignity? More so, how do we go beyond that to make this the most exciting and rewarding time of our lives?

Grace and dignity are not new to us. Grace is the ability one may possess to accept things in a manner that is calm, considerate, loving, and reflective. Dignity is one's ability to maintain a positive sense of self. Dignity means taking pride in being able to do things for ourselves, to stand up for ourselves and be independent as well. Some of us have trouble with grace and dignity without leaning on someone else for support, while others may take pleasure in being loners and using their machismo to function no matter what. Women may use the power of their inner strength in this case. Either way, the use of these two words is irreplaceable, making life without them more difficult and somewhat tenuous.

The world for most of us is a black abyss of space that needs to be explored before we find meaning and define it for ourselves, notwithstanding that some of us never get there even when we age. Life for others is mindless and just flows from day to day. For the majority, life is made up of moments that challenge the fabric of our being. Each strand of life can bring energy to our souls, making us hunger for more until we have our fill of life: learning, growing, changing continuously, being whipped up into a mass of swirling protoplasm defining and redefining our existence, authoring our own lives.

Coming of age happens to us in stages, as writer Gail Sheehy so aptly wrote in *Passages* (Random House, 1976) and psychologist and psychoanalyst Erik Erikson so methodically and exactly defined in his socioemotional development analysis. Each stage of life for an individual is predicated by some event. These events may be potty training, a first shave, a first kiss, a breaking away from home and becoming independent, buying a first home, attaining a profession, graduating college, having grandchildren or great grandchildren, and finally reaching death. I say *reaching* because this is a process in life, as is aging a part of the dying process itself. But it is the minute differences at each stage that give meaning to one's life. One has to be primed for this information, ready to grab what comes out of each experience the moment it happens. This too is a process: the way we react to things and the way we make things happen for ourselves that bring inner meaning to the aging process.

A new paradigm in aging is such that the numbers of years are used to demarcate the stages of life with respect to being young, old, and finally becoming an elder. We live in a throw-away society.

People, by the time they become old, are used up and cast aside, or so we think. No other social habitat in the world parallels the one found in our society. Elders need to be held on to, cherished and nourished for their wisdom, and to help offset that part of our society that chugs along mindlessly, not knowing, not contributing; just using up life, not giving back to it. Our elders are a great source of power and ability.

What I have learned from older people constitutes most of what I have learned during half of my life. Just think about how much one can learn from elders: our teachers; our relatives; our acquaintances; our role models; our grandparents; and so on.

More people over the age of sixty-five years are continuing to work and not retiring these days—25 percent of our population to be exact. The same percentage of people over the age of sixty-five years are reinventing themselves in schools, going back to learn new things, and gaining more knowledge to share and use for the betterment of self and society. We can age gracefully by moving with the flow and adapting to the changes, whether subtle or brazen. We can take pride in our status as seasoned individuals with knowledge to share and we can help others be successful in their own right by providing a little coaching from our perspective.

Who says you have to be old? That's really it, isn't it? We all age, some of us more slowly than others by the luck of the draw, but it happens to all of us. Being old is a state of mind. I remember a young boy I was friends with in high school. I cannot remember his name or see his face; I just remember the experience that provoked this thought. I remember his mother calling a bunch of the "boys," his friends, together telling us we would not be able to see her son again as he was dying of leukemia. This came as a shock to me and the others as well but more than that I remember thinking that he would never grow old or see old age. At the same time, I experienced something that contributed to living my own life and learned about the aging process at a very young age indeed. We all face the vicissitudes of life at one time or another along the way.

Death, which I will talk about in a later chapter, is a mystery to most all of us. We may choose to recognize it or deny it; yet, all too often little glimpses of light penetrate our psyches showing us that the thoughts are there. As a kid, I wondered what death was for my friend and whether he would be happy or sad, continue living in a different manner, and be able to guide his friends from afar.

These thoughts are still with me about others who have died since then, and thoughts about my own vulnerability and mortality still gnaw at me from time to time.

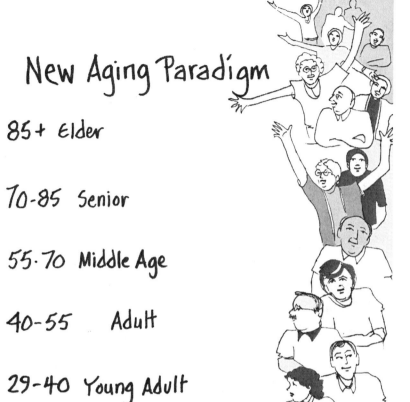

New Aging Paradigm

85+ Elder

70-85 Senior

55-70 Middle Age

40-55 Adult

29-40 Young Adult

0-29 Emerging Young Adult

In reality, we don't have to accept the fact that we are old or even aging. Being old in our society too often connotes being inept, out of touch, ignorant, poor, and incapable of functioning anymore. There are many myths, considered as ageism, that pervade our culture and that the masses still believe; but if you look at the ages of people in our world who have achieved major scientific breakthroughs, it proves that age is irrelevant. I will repeat myself here by saying that being old is a state of mind, not an aging body.

Recently, a Russian-born American economist, Leonid Hurwiz, won the Nobel Prize in Economics at age ninety years for his basic economic theory that determines when markets are working effectively. Frank Lloyd Wright was still designing houses at ninety-two years of age. George Burns, the late comic, resurrected his show-biz life at seventy-nine years and performed to the ripe old age of one hundred years. He certainly never acted as if he were old; he often appeared with two young women, both lightly clad and hanging off his arms, making jokes about sex at his age.

His humor deflected any semblance of remorse about his age or functioning at that age. If one can laugh at things then it lessens the anxiety about any pain or suffering caused by feeling something in a negative or depressive way. Humor breaks tension and this is a good way to deflect being uncomfortable about aging—make fun of yourself in light of the difficulty. I remember George Burns's comments about sex just before he died: "Sex for me, at my age, is like shooting pool with a rope!"

Making fun of oneself in the face of adversity is a true sign of maturity, acceptance, making peace with one's body, one's actions and allowing others the comfort of knowing that they too may not be alone with their unmet needs. Aging is all about acceptance. Allowing oneself permission to accept and process any transition that occurs while one ages will keep one ultimately youthful. I am fully convinced of this fact.

Writer Norman Cousins advocated the healing power of humor and laughter in his book *Anatomy of an Illness as Perceived by the Patient* (Bantam Books, New York, 1979). Acceptance is allowing oneself to heal. Cousins overcame much adversity and illness through continued laughter and making jokes about himself as well as others. Laughter, courage, and tenacity are needed to overcome any disease or situation that limits one in growing older and staying healthy doing so.

AGING WITH IDENTITY

Identity, with respect to self, starts with one's forebears. Those of us wondering how old we will live to be will just have to take a look at our grandparents and great-grandparents and extrapolate our own age at the end of our lives with respect to how long these people lived. At least 70 percent of one's longevity is tied into genetics, and 30 percent of longevity is associated with lifestyle. Wanting to live to a ripe old age, then, is an extension of how long our ancestors stuck around.

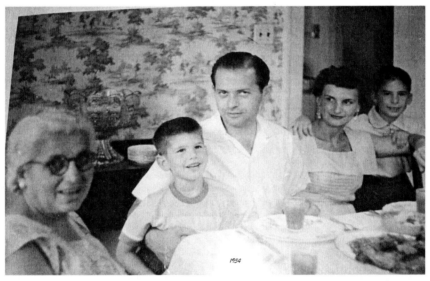

Bubbie, Brother Harvey, Dad, Mom, Me. Circa 1955

At the beginning of the twentieth century, the average age at death was around forty-seven years old. Today, the average lifespan is about seventy-eight years for men and eighty-six years for women (U.S. Census Bureau, 2004). Specifically, knowing that most of the men died young in a certain family due to heart disease should be a signal to the present generation of men in that family to work hard at maintaining a good diet, exercise regimen, state of mind, and attitude.

Eliminating negative impacts to a long life, like excessive drinking, lack of exercise, smoking, and hard drugs, is critical. Diets rich in fresh fruits and vegetables are a must. Dr. Walter Bortz, geriatrician, advocates "living like a Bushman" in order to live to be a hundred. That is, go back to eating like our ancient ancestors, who ate natural grains, berries, and other natural foods from what nature provided us at that time. Limiting red meats, animal fats, and large amounts of carbohydrates and trans fats will help preserve our bodies and keep them youthful and strong, as will taking supplements when needed and antioxidants.

Sleep is essential to living a long time, and everyone should try to at least take a cat-nap daily in order to rejuvenate the mind and body. "Beware of that poison apple" said the dwarves to Snow White. OK, she didn't listen, but her sleep preserved her youth and beauty until the guy who couldn't stay away any longer gave her a kiss on the lips, arousing her from slumber. Being intimate with another person doesn't hurt either in the quest to stay young.

Therefore, the six keys to living a long, healthy life are:

1. stimulating the mind;
2. staying social;
3. eating right;
4. getting enough rest;
5. experiencing intimacy of one sort or another; and
6. remaining ambulatory.

There is a seventh key, the lucky key I call it, which is getting out of your self. That means giving your gifts away, sharing your expertise, if you will, with someone who is less fortunate than you. This will come back to you many times in added longevity, happiness and self-satisfaction.

The U.S. Surgeon General asks that all of us exercise at least five to seven days for thirty continuous minutes. I wonder if that includes sex. This is a lot to ask when many of us work long hours and only plan to exercise on the weekends or nightly using finger exercises on the buttons of our remote controls

Real identity comes from the discovery and acknowledgment of our heritage. Many are lucky to be able to maintain long, closely knit, and communicative relationships with their families. In such cases, gleaning your history is easy. To be able to spend time with elders, listening to their stories, is a wonderful gift that we receive from and give to each other.

Looking at my own family, I have had to work hard at retrieving information for my own sense of self. I moved to the East Coast to go to college near my father's large family and then made frequent trips to visit them, to get to know my grandmother (my father's mother) and the many aunts, uncles, and cousins. This allowed them to get to know me as well. I found out that my father was born when his father was seventy-six years old! I hope I have some of my grandfather's genes. My father did not really get to know his father, as my grandfather did not speak English. With twelve brothers and sisters to compete with, being the youngest male, and not being able to communicate with his father in English, my father was at a distinct disadvantage in knowing what his father was like or in receiving direct family history to enable his own development and sense of self. Not knowing one's heritage is stifling and harmful to the psyche. Without identity one needs to forage alone in order to find out about his or her roots and family make-up.

Many years ago, I was watching a symphony in Toronto where I was visiting for a meeting. Some people came in and sat by me. They were speaking in some foreign tongue, and I listened closely enough to ascertain it was Yiddish. I interrupted them to ask if they had ever heard of my grandfather, who supposedly founded and built the first synagogue in Toronto on the property where Eaton Square now stands. The oldest of the group, a man in his seventies, said he did not know of my grandfather but did know an even older gentleman whom he took to the market every weekend. He offered to ask the older gentleman if he knew anything about my grandfather.

To preface my discussion with these strangers, my father, who was alive at the time, had told me before I went on the trip to Canada to look up my grandfather's heritage in Toronto: the synagogue which my grandfather had built at the turn of the twentieth century. I had tried to do this but no one seemed to know anything about the place, which no longer existed. It had been replaced by Eaton Center, a huge shopping complex, one of the biggest in the world.

About two days after the concert, I received a call from the man I sat next to at the symphony (I'll call him Sam). He was out of breath and very much excited with the news he was about to tell me. He kept ranting: "A miracle has happened! A miracle has happened!" I asked him to calm down and tell me of this miracle. Sam told me that on his way to the market with the old man he wanted to query, he had asked him if he knew or had heard of my grandfather. When he mentioned the name I gave him, Asher Zalig, the old man exclaimed, "That's mein uncle!" which would have made the old man my second cousin.

Sam was so enthralled at the coincidence that he immediately set up a meeting between the old man and me for the day before I was to leave, not caring about the schedule of events at my meeting. Sam was so excited that a miracle had happened that he was determined to carry out his plan no matter what.

Sam came to get me at my hotel and drove me for about an hour out of town to his home. He lived in the outskirts of Toronto in a high-rise apartment house. When I came in to the apartment, his wife, Golda, beckoned me to sit and eat. Most Jewish households of tradition never let anyone get away with coming into their home and not eating. Believe me, there were enough appetizers for a meal and a half and at least ten more people.

About ten minutes after I arrived, by which time I was completely stuffed, there came a knocking at the door. I guessed it to be the old man, but at this point I was so engrossed in appetizers I was in a state of hyperventilation and delirium! Sam went over and opened the door. I looked over toward the door expecting to see an old man, stooped over with a cane or walker, bald, feeble, and with tremors. Much to my surprise, here stood a giant of a man with a full head of white hair, built like a body builder, about six feet five inches.

I gasped in disbelief, food falling from my lips. The "old man," somewhere in his mid-eighties, had tears running down his cheeks even before the door opened, and as I stood to greet him for a formal introduction, trying to get my senses together, he literally lunged over to me, picked me up in a bear hug, squeezed the air out of me, and kissed my cheeks, my eyes, my ears, every part of my face in rapid succession, leaving nothing untouched by his lips until I was completely saturated with his tears of enthusiasm and ready to pass out.

Finally realizing the impact of his actions, the man, whose name was Harry, set me down ever so gently and handed me his handkerchief apologetically, blubbering about how wonderful it was to meet me. By this time, I was exhausted and could hardly stand up. Coming out of my state of being overwhelmed, I also realized that a small handkerchief wouldn't do the job, I needed a bath towel.

The next three hours were filled with wonder and amazement. Harry, who was in his eighties, told me incredible things about my grandfather that even my father had not known: how my grandfather brought his entire family over from Europe in order to save them from the rigors of war; how my grandfather found the family places to live; how the family traveled across the Atlantic, for weeks, in the bowels of a steamer crammed with human suffering and not enough room to exercise or hardly breathe, until they arrived in North America; and how my grandfather eventually found jobs for everyone. The trip from Europe to Canada in the steamer caught my attention. The struggles of the family to survive the trip with complete lack of dignity, amenities, food, bathroom facilities, warmth, and fresh air was enough to make anyone writhe with feelings of discomfort, empathy, and disbelief.

Comparing our own lives with those of our ancestors can bring us the satisfaction of knowing how lucky we are and the appreciation of what the older generations had to endure in order to improve the lives of their kin. This type of experience also gives us insight into the habits, the nuances, and the need for reassurance as well as love, food, and shelter—important aspects of life for everyone.

The time with Harry went by in an instant, and I had a glimpse into my family's past and a realization of the benevolence, commitment, and dedication of my grandfather as well as the history of my father's family. Benevolence—wishing to do good or being charitable (The Oxford American Desk Dictionary and Thesaurus, Second Edition, 2001)—is something that apparently ran in my family which neither I, nor my immediate family, were aware of at the time. This experience also showed me the keen memory, as if it were yesterday, my distant cousin Harry had with his recall of explicit details of his journey from

Europe as a child to the New World. Who says older people lose their memories? Not so, not this "old man."

Like millions of others, much of my family history was lost in the Holocaust. Much of the richness of our forefathers' lives with their respective families is gone forever. However, I was fortunate to meet many of my father's brothers and sisters and my grandmother on my father's side as well.

Bubbie

My "bubbie," as we called her, was a sweet and gentle woman. She was about thirty years old when my father was born. There was an obvious difference in age between her and my grandfather, but in those days, the marriages were fixed up between people and arranged by their respective parents for dowries paid out in money or goods or both. In the case of my grandmother, I do not know for sure, but my grandfather was a wealthy land baron and he could have paid a lot for the opportunity to marry my grandmother. Apparently, he bought her a farm so that they could raise their children in peace and with their own food.

My father grew up in an Orthodox Jewish home on a farm in Gibsonia, Pennsylvania. My bubbie told me a story about my dad being chased by a goose across the farm until she could get to the screaming beast and beat it away with a broom. I had to laugh, thinking that my dad was subject to an attack by a goose, until my grandmother told me how fierce these animals were and how geese were actually the watchdogs on the farm. My grandmother seemed such a gentle woman; who would have thought that she could have been the perpetrator of such an act? But she did it.

There were times when I just wanted to melt into my grandmother's arms. Her touch was as soft as down, and the way she stroked the back of my hand was soothing and peaceful to the point of being mesmerizing. I visited her in her later years of her life, when she would go out of her way to make me potato blintzes or other delicious things to eat at the expense of resting or enjoying other things she liked to do. But it seemed that above all, this cooking ritual was her greatest pleasure and the one and only gift she could give me without conditions or expectations on anyone's part.

She lived in the Jewish Home for the Aged just outside Pittsburgh, Pennsylvania in her last years of life, where she had a small apartment and hot plate to cook on. I used to visit her while I was in college about an hour or so from where she lived. I tried to make it there about once a month, just to get my fix of good Jewish cooking. She was a gift sent from heaven. Every time I left, I had tears in my eyes thinking that I might not see her again. Then, one day, it happened without warning. She was gone and so was that part of my life. I feel the loss to this day but carry fond memories I have of her close to my heart. I know that I can just look them up any time I get into a space where I want or need to remember the good and wonderful feelings of unconditional love, warmth, and care she gave to me.

This is what my Bubbie brought to me in those moments when I thought of nothing else but my stomach and the joy of bringing her pleasure with my company. I have an old, crinkled Polaroid picture of her in her nineties that brings back a surge of good feelings when I look at it. I think it is good to have reminders of people and things that bring these types of feelings to the fore from time to time. I find it interesting that we can look back on our relationships with elders, picking through the many feelings that we have for them and then learning from those feelings what it was that they gave us in the short time that we may have spent with them. It lets us know what precious role we may someday play for our younger generations.

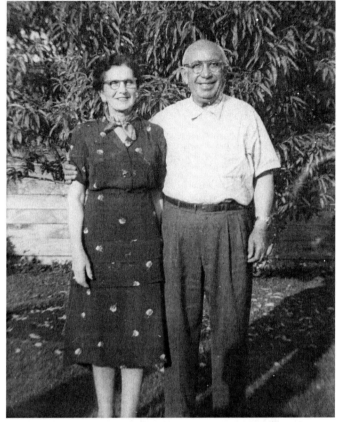

Nani and Pappa (Evelyn and Jacob Wilks)

Nani

My grandmother on my mother's side is a different story. She was fortunate to immigrate, at a young age, to America. I remember one story about her life that she told me only once. In the beginning of World War I, my grandmother found herself married at the age of about fifteen years and subsequently traipsing through the battlefield trying to take care of her Austro-Hungarian soldier husband in the trenches, until he was killed. She tried to look after him by finding scraps of food for him to eat and cigar butts for him to smoke.

After his death, she returned to her village, where the elders asked her to go to the castle of Emperor Franz Josef I of Austria, who was in his eighties at the time, to try and beg for food for their starving village. The emperor had an eye for beauty, keeping house with numerous mistresses, each in her own castle. My grandmother was young, quite beautiful, impressionable, willing, and fragile. She went to the emperor's main castle in Vienna without a word and without controversy. Nani, as we called her, spent many months in the emperor's castle as a concubine, which she never really disclosed or admitted to any in the family, except to me. She emerged, from time to time, with a parchment, sealed with a large red, royal seal, instructing the stockade to release food to her village. She was a hero in her day, but because the story was so painful to recall she found it too difficult to discuss it or any other part of her Eastern European heritage.

I believe she also lost a baby during that young part of her life but never spoke of this tragedy. I asked her if she still had any of those particular pieces of parchment with the big red seal on them, but much to my chagrin and everyone else's, she did not. This paper would have been a wonderful family heirloom as well as a great part of the history of the world in that era. Lost history is what we have when our elders do not communicate their lives to us in some way. It is up to us to glean as much as we can in order to relay this information to others, so that all of us can learn from each other.

I always wondered why my grandmother focused most of her life on cooking and encouraging us to eat whenever we arrived to visit. Of course, Nani was of Jewish heritage, so I shouldn't have thought twice about it. My mother's refrigerator was always filled, too, with so much that one could not find anything within the confines of this minisupermarket even if it was right in front of their nose. The trauma of going hungry at a young age leaves its mark and can carry over to future generations with its effects. My mother never went hungry, but Nani had experienced the pangs of hunger and the pain of not having enough to eat many a time. Finishing the food on one's plate was mandatory and essential. It wasn't worth suffering the consequences: a verbal tongue lashing with comments relating to all of the starving people in the world, mostly in Poland or China, who were not as lucky as we were to have food to eat any time we wanted it. "Now eat up!" It is a wonder that I did not end up a casualty of excess weight. I am now writing a historical novel based on my grandmother's life. I think her story should be told, even in a fictionalized way. This story will give others insight into lost history and maybe it will be the spark for them to investigate their own elders' history.

My grandfather on my mother's side, Jacob or Pappa as we called him, was a taciturn individual and provoked fear in people just from his looks. But, once you got to know him, he was a loving, caring, gentle giant of a man. I did not know much about him because he died at age fifty-seven, when I was only twelve years old. I remember my parents telling me that he went on a long trip somewhere and would not return. I cried for days even though I had no idea of the permanence of the loss.

I do know that he ran a grocery store in Carnegie, Pennsylvania, with my Nani. They would now and then send my mother to the butcher, by bus, to buy a live turtle and subsequently, have it butchered so that my Nani could make turtle soup for the customers in the restaurant part of their grocery store. My mother told me harrowing stories about how she would buy the turtle, have it butchered, wrapped, and then take the bus back to the grocery/restaurant feeling the turtle wriggle in her arms. She told me that she would let out a blood-curdling scream, stopping the bus in its tracks. The driver would ask her to leave the bus, and she would have to make her way on foot back to the grocery in time for my grandmother to cook the turtle soup. After my Nani made the soup, mother told me that the turtle continued to swim in the soup for a while longer. She took delight in watching the faces of customers choke at the sight of the turtle doing the backstroke.

I tell these few memorable stories because they illustrate the history of the family. Family stories are an integral part of a person's makeup, personality, and identity. We are the sum total of all our experiences in life, and these acts and subsequent reactions to change are what cause us to think in specific ways and to develop certain mannerisms and characteristics. As unpredictable as events are in one's life, they mold the thinking and the identity of not only the people having them but future generations that follow as well.

My mother, being an only child, gleaned a great deal from my Nani. My mother's extraordinary cooking skills and her hoarding behavior with food were traits that she learned from her mother, who in turn, had experiences in her lifetime that had etched a path for my Nani to follow as part of her everyday existence. The sense of survival in conjunction with the need to overcome the vicissitudes in one's life is essential human nature—hardwiring each and every one of us to adapt to change and survive.

Our identities come from the harvesting of the experiences we allow ourselves to absorb and our ability to hone a sense of self-awareness of what we have or will become as a result of these experiences. A good majority of personality issues comes from aberrant experiences that are misabsorbed in one's psyche, leading to a lack of self-awareness and to self-doubt. This amoeboid response ultimately affects our ability to form an identity vis-à-vis our heritage and family attributes. Basically, these may be identified with characteristics related to one's family history. It must be assumed, then, that without identity there is no sense of self.

The effects of dementia can bring on similar effects and loss of one's identity, as can old age itself. Identity of self with relation to aging should be a smooth transition, almost seamless in its process and subtle in its ability to form the final product, an elder. Most elders function in a healthy manner. Only about 5 percent of elders over the age of eighty-five find themselves captive in skilled nursing facilities because they cannot care for themselves. People eighty-five years and over are the fastest growing cohort of individuals in our day. At least 10 percent of these elders have children over the age of sixty-five!

The fact that people in today's world are living longer gives families the opportunity to get to know each other far better than those of us whose ancestors died at younger ages. Consistently, women live longer than men in our society. This means that most of us have had a chance to know the women in our families somewhat better, but no matter how one may look at family dynamics, the more information we learn from each other about family history and the lives of those who preceded us, the greater the chance to know more about ourselves and why we are who we are today.

Knowing my second cousin Harry, the "old man," gave me insight into my father and his father before him. Knowing my grandmothers gave me much insight into learning about myself as well. When I was a child, both my parents worked and my grandparents, on my mother's side, were the ones who watched over me. I have many fond memories of the way they treated me, allowing me to develop a sense of self with respect to my family heritage. The nights I spent on my grandparents' couch, with their dining room chairs, all six of them, backed up against the edge of the couch, towels spread on the backs of the chairs to block my view from the only TV set in the apartment, are wonderful remembrances for me.

I used to sneak looks between the towels at wrestling, which my grandfather was passionate about, when I should have been sleeping. But who could sleep with that noise? I saw Mr. Moto and Gorgeous

George with his flowing locks, to name a couple of the wrestlers, get slammed to the mat or scream out in a sleeper-hold many a time until they slumped into a lifeless mass. I watched with amazement and trepidation about who was going to win and who was the better showman, night after night until I was lulled to sleep by the cheers of the audience and my grandparents. I know that my grandparents did not want me to learn about violence at such a young age, but to them this was entertainment. They rarely ever went out because they were taking care of me. Several years later, my brother came on the scene, creating more work for both of them. The addition of my brother meant there was less room on the couch, and it became more difficult for me to get in my wrestling fix unless I actually started wrestling with my brother. Much to my chagrin, my grandfather put an end to this quickly with one of his stern looks and the shake of his index finger.

There were occasions, maybe three or four per week, when I spent hours in my grandfather's basement playing in his giant rolltop desk. The basement in the apartment house was like a maze, filled with incredible antiques, old furniture, dusty old books, boxes holding secrets of the past, skeleton keys by the pound, and even a Winchester rifle from the Civil War. I wonder whatever happened to all that stuff, especially the rifle, which was my favorite thing to hold and admire. I used to pretend I was in the cavalry waiting for the attack of wild Indians. The handle was bronze with fancy engraving on it, and it had a blue barrel with a wonderfully carved wooden stock. It was a real prize. I think my grandmother sold it when my grandfather died.

Lost memories—except in my own mind, which is an attic filled with cluttered scenes from my childhood that brought me much joy, mystery, and lots of fun at the time. Both my grandparents, each in their own way, taught me manners, self-respect, discipline, and commitment through their persistent reminders of how to behave and when to adhere to strict standards and mores.

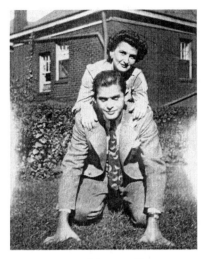

Betty and Irving Shapira Circa 1940's

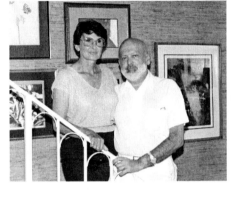

Betty and Irving Shapira Circa 1980

I remember just a few of my childhood friends. We all used to play army, jumping walls, climbing trees, and building lookouts in the walnut trees, which were vestiges of the large orchards of the past filling the San Fernando Valley with its many produce trees of fruits and nuts. We even dug underground forts and divided ourselves into teams, one against the other. Sometimes I would hide and never be found. By the time I came out of hiding, it was dark outside, and the rest of the gang were in their homes eating dinner or doing their homework. I was alone with my own thoughts.

Pep

My uncle Morris, or Uncle Pep, as we called him, was a decorated hero of World War II. I heard many stories about him from my father, and I wanted to be like him. He won a Silver Star at the Battle of the Bulge in Germany. He held off an entire battalion of Germans with a machine gun, while all his own troops were killed. He suffered frostbite on both feet and had trouble with them the rest of his life.

On meeting him, you would not expect this soft-spoken gentleman to have done what he did as a young man. Uncle Pep worked for the IRS as a collection agent but spent the majority of his time fixing watches. Later in his life, when I was visiting from college, I used to watch him put on his magnifying glasses and use his tweezers to manipulate the innards of fine watch mechanisms.

My father told me that my uncle Pep had been his protector. Pep was constantly squeezing two small rubber balls in the palms of his hands. He subsequently had a grip like iron because of this exercise. One would never know it looking at this man with his gentle handshake, but he could, with one squeeze, easily break the neck of a man twice his size.

Uncle Pep told me once that he used to shove his foot in the door when he was greeted by people who found out he was an IRS agent and was there to collect back taxes. I guess because of his frostbite, the slamming of the door on his feet went unnoticed. Either that or he had steel plating in his shoes as well.

Uncle Pep taught me patience and kindness. He was humble yet demonstrative. His language was full of lessons as he taught one the rules of life from his perspective. "Don't do unto others what they might do unto you" was his philosophy. Pep was indeed a gentle giant.

LEAH AND JOE

Each one of my father's family members, whom I had the pleasure to meet, taught me something of value, something I could absorb and use in my life both to help me and eventually to help others.

My aunt Leah, my father's younger sister, is a very strong woman. She and her husband, my uncle Joe, owned a bar and restaurant in

Pittsburgh, Pennsylvania. Aunt Leah had three boys, Arnie, Norman, and David, all of whom became doctors and all of whom I looked at as my own brothers. She encouraged these boys from the get-go, as she did me. I let myself learn from her mothering of my cousins since I was away from home and the influence of my own mother for so long. Aunt Leah gave me the gift of listening. I could go to her at any time, and she would make the time to listen to me in a nonjudgmental sort of way, even though she was most opinionated about how her boys were to turn out.

My uncle Joe was a hard-working man, committed to his family and his restaurant and always making time to encourage me, nurture me, and take care of me. I never went hungry when I came to visit his restaurant or their home. Both of these fine people were like second parents to me, and I owe them much gratitude for their care and kindness to me while I was a student in their midst. I remember those pastrami sandwiches Joe made for me like it was yesterday. My mouth waters as I think of them!

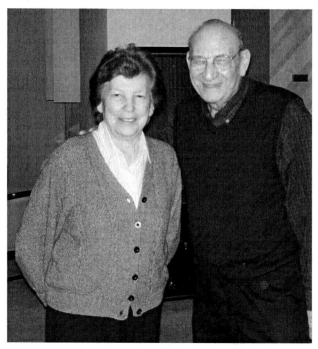

Aunt Leah and Uncle Joe Broudy

Fanny and Saul

My aunt Fanny, my father's eldest sister, was a real one-of-a kind person. She was an Orthodox Jew (one of the few remaining family members who still practiced this form of Judaism), and she lived with two sets of dishes and all the rules and regulations that went along with what she considered the official religion. Aunt Fanny and her husband, Uncle Saul, a kosher butcher, allowed me to live in their attic while I attended graduate school one year. Their house was a block from the Pittsburgh Zoo, and every night I was serenaded. I could hear the roar of the lions, shrills of the monkeys, squawking of the parrots, trumpeting of the elephants, and more. I knew when it was feeding time for the animals and when they were in estrus, ready to mate. I used to fantasize about being in deepest, darkest Africa where I was alone in the jungle with all these beasts at night.

Sometimes those nights were a very frightening proposition for me and created the desire for some kind of a sedative in order to get some sleep amidst the commotion across the street. These are memories from the late sixties—and to think that I didn't even need drugs for this kind of trip! Of course, it is said that if you remember the sixties, it really did not happen for you, but for me it did. The strange experiences were real. I did not use drugs, but maybe I should have since I was living with people who were totally the antithesis of what I was all about. Their habits seemed crazy, such as not eating meat products with dairy, including hearing strange animal noises on cue every night for hours on end. There were reasons for this I am sure, but I did not know what they were for at the time?

My aunt Fannie's daughter, Diane, also lived in the house. She was like the big sister I never had. At times, I found her friendship most comforting, but she always had a word for me about how I should run my life, which added to my level of frustration. I was grateful to her for translating the orthodox rituals for me and keeping me on the straight and narrow track in the house so as not to cross any lines I did not understand. I also was a confidant for Diane, listening to her for hours on end about her frustrations in life and living at home. I had some terrific experiences living with my father's relatives. Experiences I would not trade for anything.

I remember one night specifically, when I was studying away into all hours of the night in my attic bedroom, even forgetting to eat, I suddenly realized the emptiness of my stomach and how very hungry I had become. I did not want to disturb any of my aunt's kitchen rituals by raiding the refrigerator and interfering with her religious convictions or waking up the family, so I walked down to the corner convenience store and bought myself a ham sandwich no less, taking it back to my small, semi-lit attic room about midnight. Well, needless to say, God struck me down that night disabling me for the next several days with a severe stomach ache, nausea, and vomiting. I knew right there I was going to die a horrible and unforgivable death! I also realized that at that point I should not have tempted fate by bringing nonkosher food into a kosher house, especially a ham sandwich. That was the only time. One only does foolish things once, and the lesson is learned.

I moved out right after that experience, just in case I got hungry in the night again sometime in the future. I never told my aunt the reason for the move, even though she kept questioning me about the decision to move from a free room to one that I had to pay for with my meager means. My aunt knew I was broke, and I think she knew somehow what I had done. She had a direct line to God; I was and still am convinced of it.

My aunt Fanny was a kind and generous person. She was also very intuitive and dedicated to her principles. If you lived in her home, you were bound to follow these principles or be cursed. I found out first hand. Aunt Fanny always had an ear for me. From her I learned values, conviction, strength, religion, love and empathy. She died many years later of cancer but never let on how much pain she was in at the time. I felt so helpless watching her die. In the end, she only had concerns for me as if I were one of her children. To this day, I think I really was her surrogate. She never let me go without anything. Fanny always had a lesson to teach and a caring hand and bent ear for listening. She taught me about the meaning of empathy with the way she lived her life. She was a real peach of a gal.

Aunt Fannie's husband, Uncle Saul, was a good provider and made sure that I lacked for nothing as well, but he was quiet, religious, stern, and from the old school. In the long run, his mannerisms would win out and at some point in time I could really appreciate his generosity and "soft-touch" kind of heart. I think I learned from him that one cannot always express what one is feeling; however, those feelings might come out through actions rather than words.

SAUL

My father's oldest brother, Saul, was an attorney and the only one of my grandmother's children who had the fortune to go to college and finish with a degree. His hobby was reading the dictionary to classical music! "Try it, you'll like," he would say to me. I found it easier to learn words while listening to music, and this became the basis for my studying ritual, learning with a beat! My goal had always been to be a scholar.

I felt humbled in front of my uncle Saul because of what he had achieved and because he knew so much about life, nature, politics, and just about anything else that was going on in the world. He was well read and became the head of his father-in-law's food market chain at a young age and very wealthy at the same time. All of his children, David, Danny, Ralph, and Edie, became successful professionals in their own right.

I found a common theme running deep among my family: the need for knowledge in the form of a formal education and the need to make something of oneself. This provoked a sense of pride, I felt, in the uncles and aunts toward their children, and I wanted this for myself, yet never quite receiving it or hearing this type of pride from my own parents until many years after the fact.

My observation of these family principles fueled my own sense of determination to make something of myself so that my parents would eventually be proud of me, which would allow me to feel they accepted me. I realize now, at this earlier stage of my life, that I was searching for my own sense of self—who I was; what I was to become. I was grabbing at the things my family members taught me about life, themselves, the way they treated their own children, and their perceptions about the world around us.

Unbeknownst to me at the time, these values were the basis for my ability to overcome great obstacles in the future. I realize now that I have those innate parts of my relatives inside me to thank for my fortitude, vision, tenacity, and success.

> *In the stillness of night Wisdom came and stood by my bed. She gazed upon me like a tender mother and wiped away my tears, and said: "I have heard the cry of your spirit and I am come to comfort it. Open your heart to me and I shall fill it with light. Ask of me and I shall show you the way of truth." And I said: "Who am I, Wisdom, and how came I to this frightening place? And these words composed by desire and sung by delight, what are they? What are these conclusions, grievous and joyous, that embraces my spirit and envelops my heart? And those eyes which look at me seeing into my depths and fleeing from my sorrows? And those voices mourning my days and chanting my littleness, what are they? What is this youth that plays with my desires and mocks at my longings, forgetful of yesterday's deeds, rejoicing in paltry things of the moment, scornful of the morrow's coming? What is this world that leads me whither I know not, standing with me in despising? And this earth that opens wide its mouth to swallow bodies and lets evil things to dwell on its breast?" ... And she answered: "It is that which draws your spirit. It is that which you see and makes you to give rather than receive.*

It is that thing you feel when hands are stretched forth from your depths to clasp it to your depths. It is that which the body reckons a trial and the spirit a bounty. It is the link between joy and sorrow. It is all that you perceive hidden and know unknown and hear silent. It is a force that begins in the holy of holies of your being and ends in that place beyond your visions."

—Kahlil Gibran, A Visit From Wisdom,
A Tear and A Smile

Seeking to understand myself in relation to my family, my teachers, and the world around me was a hidden quest. The quoted poem by Gibran illustrates a process. It is a process of questioning that which we learn, that which we observe, and that which questions each of us as we try to understand our importance in the scheme of things. The process is one that should continue through life so that we can benchmark our desires in relation to those things we have accomplished and those things yet to be accomplished.

For me, at this time in my life, I was just beginning to understand family dynamics, perhaps because I was growing older and accumulating wisdom. Having some identity now gave me the advantage of understanding my roots, thus giving me direction for future endeavors.

The importance of understanding your identity cannot be overstated because it allows you the opportunity to benchmark and validate your life in the scheme of things. Ask yourself how you are doing and if you are on the right path. Compare yourself to your family members and gauge for yourself how far you have come. Set goals now for your future and plan for change.

What I learned from the older people I discussed in this chapter, who never acted their age, formed the basis for what I intended to accomplish in my life: acquiring knowledge; understanding life around me; appreciating nature and all that it brings to us; and mastering skills that would allow me to provide a living and a life's work for myself. Understanding the child within and the ability to nurture this child would keep me young all of my life and provide me with the sense of wonder one needs to appreciate new things and cherish those things that have come and gone.

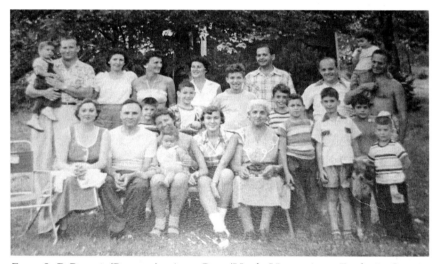

From L-R Row 1 (Bottom): Aunt Rose/Uncle Harry, Aunt Freda & Cousin Edie, Cousin Rhoda, Bubbie, Cousin Norman, Me, Cousin Ralph, Cousin Mike. From L-R Row 2 (Top): Uncle Joe & Cousin David, Aunt Leah, Mom, Brother Harvey, Cousin Arnie, Aunt Pearl, Cousin David, Dad, Cousin Danny, Uncle Pep, Uncle Saul & Cousin Barbara. Circa 1955

Chapter 2

When the Music Changes, So Does the Dance

MAKING CHANGES

Two roads diverged in a yellow wood,
And sorry I could not travel both
And be one traveler, long I stood
And looked down one as far as I could
To where it bent in the undergrowth;

Then took the other, as just as fair,
And having perhaps the better claim,
Though as for that the passing there
Had worn them really about the same,
And both that morning equally lay

In leaves no step had trodden black,
Oh, I kept the first for another day!
Yet knowing how way leads on to way,
I doubted if I should ever come back.
I shall be telling this with a sigh

Somewhere ages and ages hence:
Two roads diverged in a wood, and I—

Dr. Eric Z. Shapira, DDS, MA, MHA

> *I took the one less traveled by,*
> *And that has made all the difference.*
>
> —Robert Frost, American poet, "The Road Not Taken"

What I have learned from older people about change is that it is not only inevitable, but should be embraced with fervor. Life is all about change and the process of change, which in turn involves making choices. Without change there would be stagnancy, malaise, boredom, depression, sameness, and repetition. In a world with these characteristics there would be no motivation for new life, invention, fullness of thought, and zest for living. The ability to make choices regarding our lives, our livelihoods, and our thinking gives us the ability to make transitions in a free and unrestricted manner.

"Transition times are times of self-renewal" according to consultant and lecturer, formerly a professor of English, William Bridges, PhD, author of the book *Transitions* (Perseus Books, 1973). Statistics have shown that Americans change professions or jobs at least seven times in a lifetime. This is an amazing statistic when you think about it. I am sure there are those who are happy doing what they do on a daily basis, but without the high percentage of people who do change, there might not be any real progress in our society.

I can recall some of the many jobs I have had in my lifetime: administrative assistant, screw sorter for a construction company, soda jerk, gas station attendant, screen maker for windows, demolition for a construction company, dump truck driver, bar tender, ticket-taker at the movies, bookstore clerk, dental assistant, associate dentist, dentist, gerontologist, teacher, sculptor, watercolorist, and educator. These are just some of the jobs I received pay for along the way. There were many volunteer jobs in between these jobs that filled voids in my life and gave meaning to my life as well. Many people look at these change periods in their lifetimes as times of crisis, but in fact, they are part of the normal ebb and flow of our rhythms blending our internal chemicals, charging them into action and leading to subsequent productive output. Without our normal circadian rhythms, accumulating daily, our cycles of energy would not allow us to renew ourselves in the face of change with maximum flexibility and strength.

The baby-boomer generation is now approaching an age that will classify them as older individuals. This is the largest, most educated, wealthiest, and most productive group of individuals in the history of America, or the world, as a matter of fact. As of the year 2012, according to the U.S. Census Bureau, approximately 25 percent of the population will be above the age of sixty-five, and 25 percent of these people will still have the desire to be working; if not in their present jobs, then at new ones that will have been the result of self-renewal, change, and subsequent transition.

Sir Isaac Newton, the renowned scientist, codified several laws of nature. One of those laws stated that for every action, there is an equal and opposite reaction. You might remember the first time a wrong deed was discovered by a parent. Our parents' natural reaction to finding out that something was not right led to a stern scolding, punishment, or maybe both. Sometimes a long lecture accompanied the parental intrusion in order to teach a lesson of life. I remember when I was a child my father told me, "Clean your room." He came back a few hours later, looked in the room, and said, "You didn't hear me, son. I told you to clean up your room!" I responded with, "I heard you, Dad; I just didn't listen to you." I only said that once in my life! This type of situation follows us as we age. In our quests to find happiness we tend to have these ebbs and flows of action and then reaction to situations that reflect our desire or our response to change.

There is also the principle of evolutionary change. Over a million years ago, early humans were conscious of themselves as an integral part of the whole—that is, part of the environment in which they lived. They were hunters and gatherers, and they survived only if they respected the world in which they lived. Those were hard times for those individuals. The hard times of the past have been translated into the difficult times of the present, in which we all struggle to survive and live a happy and productive life. It seems to be all relative. Today, the extent of our hunting and gathering, for the most part, is going to the supermarket and making choices about what we like to eat or what we need to get by on for the next week. Our choices are vast, and our lives are much more complicated than the lives of our Stone Age brothers and sisters were. Evolutionary changes came about with the discovery of fire, clothing, tools, and other discoveries that made life more convenient. As these things became more sophisticated in the scheme of things, mankind evolved to having an easier time with surviving and getting on in life.

According to Richard Leakey, world-famous archaeologist, humans evolved from a life of hunting and gathering to one of farming about ten thousand years ago. At this juncture, man's instincts changed from a warlike attitude to a more sedentary way of life as farmers.

Looking into our past, no matter how far back, gives us insight into our future. Coupled with our own identity is our ability to make choices that will ultimately take us in the direction of least resistance. At least we hope so. This is a natural law and one which might help us understand our ancestors as well as ourselves. But, hopefully, by combining our own personal history within the family and then placing ourselves on the family map or genogram, we can make predictions about why we are who we are, why we act the way we do, and possibly predict what we might become in the future.

I know that my father did not finish college. In fact, it was extremely difficult for him to even go to school, since he was forced to work and fend for himself at a young age. However, he wanted me to go to college and make something of myself. I had the opportunity to achieve, with my parents' help. I could have predicted this scenario if I had taken the time and effort to understand where my father came from; that is, what my father went through in his life growing up and his motivations for doing what he did. I think we all want the best for our children and hope that they have it better than we do. In some ways, this has created a society that is somewhat lazy and resistant to change.

The new generations have had it too easy: growing up with cell phones, computers, and all the bells and whistles of the electronic age. Some of the boomers, whose cohorts may have created or invented these things, may still be in the dark ages about electronic devices, but even worse off are our parents, the elders in our society. Unless they are extremely motivated, they are unable to work or understand a computer or use a cell phone to save their lives. However, because so many of us depend upon the modern conveniences that are available to us both inexpensively and ubiquitously, many older individuals are now changing with the times and are taking classes to learn how to use this modern equipment as well as other subjects that they might not otherwise have had the time to learn while supporting a family.

Each time we take on something new, it is a new chapter in our life. Each time we change the way we do something, learn a new piece of information, or understand a new piece of our own puzzle, we transition and change. We evolve into a new human with abilities and ideas that keep us from stagnating. Keeping one's mind active, learning new things, and being social take on a new meaning when one might think that he or she is at the end of the line.

Life is about change: the incorporation of our ancestral identity and the inevitable will to memorialize ourselves by producing offspring who can carry on the traditions we have brought forward to them. However, change is not all about external transformation and transition; change is about internal transformation as well. For example, one can change jobs but must take on a different mindset when approaching the new job with fervor and gusto.

I remember working as a soda jerk in an ice cream parlor when I was a teenager. I could not tolerate my boss. The man was tough as nails, and much of the time he grimaced and looked around with what seemed to me to be a fiendish gaze. He had a way about him that was akin to a dictator barking commands. He seemed quite mean and overly fussy about everything. I guess today he would be classified as a micromanager. There wasn't one thing that I did that was free from the boss's comments or his watchful eye. He was constantly on me to make things perfect.

In the parlor, there were about twenty milkshake machines. Every time someone made a milkshake, I was called upon to get up on the counter and clean the large twenty-five foot mirror behind the machines. The boss even climbed up on the counter with me to show me how to clean the mirror the "right way" one day. While he was lecturing me about how to clean the glass, I became distracted from his lecture when I noticed on his arm a series of small, blue, tattooed numbers. When I went home that evening I told my mother about the experience and my observation, asking her if the numbers on my boss's arm were of significance. It was then that I learned the intricate details of the Holocaust in Europe.

This man was a *survivor*.

I had judged my boss harshly until that evening. When I learned about the significance of those numbers, which transported the boss into a different time and place some twenty to twenty-five years earlier, my perception of his life and my entire perspective about the man, the job, and the way he treated me changed in a single moment. I tried to understand what he had been through and the extent of the hardship on both him and his wife as well, but I sensed at the time that my understanding of his life was not really possible. I could only accept the fact that I was the one that needed the transformation of my thinking into a positive outlook in order to cope with my own judgment about the boss. I realized many years later that this man's discipline was his way of telling me that he cared about me. I also realized that this discipline probably kept him alive during his time of incarceration and stress. He wanted me to succeed, to survive, and to be perfect in every way. I know this now because I saw the same or similar behavior coming from my father toward me many times.

His Holiness the Dalai Lama has made clear the importance of making a sustained effort in bringing about real inner transformation and change with respect to doing a job or learning something new. His Holiness has stressed that all transformation is a gradual process and requires "positive affirmations" to discover one's "inner child." I think the key to staying youthful is never letting go of the vision of one's inner child. The inner child in all of us is a nascent truth, a joyous spirit, and a sometimes rebellious nymph that sparks our curiosity and mischievousness.

The state of youthfulness maintains all of these innocent properties. The psychologist Erik Erickson said that the sense of basic trust is by far one of the first of the components of mental health to develop in life. A sense of autonomous will is the second, and a sense of initiative is third. The birthing process brings forth a new dimension from one environment to another. The change is significant, and the properties of strength or weakness, internally, come from the formation of a new and struggling organism.

I am reminded of the story of the chrysalis hanging from the branch of a tree that I learned from a person of great intuition and empathy, my own counselor at a time of life that was most difficult for me. It was a time of great change and anguish, which I will discuss later in this book. Change is a gift of life for the lowly caterpillar as it metamorphoses in keeping with its own aging process. As it moves and squirms around, the animal inside the chrysalis is trying desperately to free itself from the confines of its exterior straitjacket of sorts. If someone cuts it free at any time before it is ready to ascend out of the cocoon by itself, the animal will die.

The reason behind this is simple and pure. The animal must struggle to set itself free, and during this time, the butterfly gathers strength, developing its muscles, so that when it does break free it will be able to fly and feed itself for survival. If the butterfly is freed by some other source it will not be able to fly and will subsequently die of starvation. This inner strength then is what Erickson is alluding to in his explanation of the human life cycle.

I like to cite these principles as factors in the actions of my childhood boss. My boss probably kept his innate, inner child locked deep within for who knows how long, while he underwent the most horrific of experiences one could possibly imagine, but keeping his inner child alive all the while. My boss's struggle to be free again was sustained by his ability to maintain some form of mental health, inner strength, and the will to survive. My newfound respect for my boss only strengthened my own perceptions of living life with tenacity, curiosity, and a positive mental attitude, as well as struggling to be free. Free of what, at the time, I was not sure, but possibly it was to be free from judging another human being.

Looking back now with a jaundiced eye gives me great perspective about the passing of time, experiences I had, regrets I still ponder, and my ability to cope and adapt in the face of it all. This was a great lesson in life for me, and a wonderful realization of how far I have evolved as a caring, empathic human being as well. Consider some of your own stories that parallel this one.

CAN AGE MAKE US CHANGE?

Being old or older does not mean we are less able to change. The will to change comes from within and may be stimulated by an event, a thought, a caring friend, a need to change or a reaction to an event. I have an older friend named Mel who is about eighty-eight years young. He is a widower after some fifty years of marriage. I say young, because he was still playing tennis, had a younger girlfriend and an active sex life, as well as an active mind the last time we met.

Mel loved to putter around in his garden, planting vegetables, and he demonstrated his pride by showing them off when these herbaceous plants came to fruition by saying something like, "My squash is the best in the county, and you can't buy anything like this anywhere." Mel still played golf and had already gone through several knee and hip replacements. He still got around driving his own car to visit friends, volunteered in the local hospital several days a week, and went out on dates. Mel, as it turned out, was a true lady's man, and a Renaissance man. He was a fine artist and inventor, coming up with his last interesting concoction while in his late seventies: a solid fuel fire starter made from wax and scrap plastic.

One day, I received a call from Mel's daughter, who told me she needed my help. When I asked if all was OK, she replied that, in a very short time span, Mel had changed. Mel had sold his house, where he and his family lived for over forty years, in two days and moved to a town about thirty miles from his home to live in a senior residence. Something fishy was going on, but I couldn't tell what.

Mel's daughter told me that he was depressed and asked if I would speak to him. When I called to question him about things, Mel told me about selling his home and the remorse he felt about doing so. He said, "I possibly made a mistake." He was now living in a senior residence where he was provided three square meals a day and there were others of his ilk to keep him company and share his anguish. These people all had their stories.

Was Mel's change due to a conscious choice or was it ruled by his unconscious mind? Was his choice made when he was not in his right state of mind? Did his girlfriend twist his arm? These things remained to be seen.

Mel was obviously depressed and taking a lot of different medicines for arthritis, for hip pain, and for who knew what. Some of the drugs he was taking were leftover medications that his deceased wife had been taking for her illness. There were many bottles of medicines that Mel was not familiar with, but he took them anyway thinking they would help.

Drug interactions can affect the way one thinks and can cause changes in both mental decision-making processes and subsequent reactions, such as this kind of aberrant thinking. Mel was taken off his medication, with my recommendation to do so, and made a one hundred and eighty degree turnaround. This kind of change was for the better; however, Mel's sale of his home and his subsequent move were irreversible.

The lesson here is one of unguided use of medication. If depression strikes older people, it is sometimes difficult to discern what drugs they should take, how much to take, when to take the medication, and when to stop the drugs. One must first determine the origin of the depression and the level of cerebral chemicals that help control our functional moods and thinking processes. The combination of drugs can also cause the depression itself.

This group of emotionally fragile people may go unsupervised as well, which can only exacerbate the situation. Making any kind of important decisions should be delayed until thinking abilities can be assessed. Depression can alter our ability to think clearly and rationally. I find that most people, when becoming hyperemotional to the point of being in a depressed state, often cannot make a rational decision. Irrationality breeds lack of clarity. Lack of clarity tends to leave people in confused states and sometimes helpless, even bordering on suicide.

Age does not necessarily have anything to do with being depressed, but it may, depending upon the circumstances. Symptoms and conditions associated with psychological stress are: illness and death; being alone; feeling isolated; financial inadequacy; or feeling not useful. These are a few of the precipitators of depression in the later stages of life. Under stress, many people, regardless of age, may not be able to make adequate decisions.

Viktor Frankl, noted psychiatrist and neurologist, who spent several years of his life in various concentration camps during World War II, expounded on these theories of existential philosophy, rationalizing the reasons for living. These theories came about when he set up suicide watches for people entering the concentration camps who were overtaken with severe stress and could not cope with being there. Immediate depression set in and so did ideas of suicide. To this end, it was necessary to have each individual look toward what was good in life, what meanings they could find in all the pain and suffering they were experiencing.

Dr. Frankl wrote his famous book in 1946, *Man's Search for Meaning* (Simon and Shuster, 1962) which discussed how he, as a concentration camp survivor, kept positive thoughts in the face of adversity. Dr. Frankl had an escape mechanism that he designed in his own head, whereby he would go outside and lecture to no one about psychiatric theory. In this act alone, Dr. Frankl found meaning and formulated some of his most famous teachings to help others.

I have found the same holds true in helping others, such as suggesting to my clients that in getting out of ourselves, we allow people the opportunity to realize their gifts. This act forces a subtle change in a person's inner self. In turn, this change may not be a recognizable change. It is clandestine and takes over your entire being; much like ivy plants growing and sticking to the sides of a building or a tree. The plants continue to envelop the structure until the structure is unrecognizable in its original state. This is how this type of change works with people who show depression and dissatisfaction with their lives. "No one knows what gifts they have until they give them away," is a motto I have adopted over the years of learning firsthand what it means.

One of my clients, who came to see me in a state of stress and frustration as well as depression, was so wrapped up in herself that she could not see the forest for the trees. She was suicidal several times during my initial year of doing geriatric counseling with her and as I monitored her mental processes, for which she had no plan, I encouraged her to uncover some of her fears, stress inducers, and concerns. After getting her to consent to help others in the local hospital by reading to them, or volunteering in various groups in the community, this woman, who I will call Georgia, started climbing out of her doldrums. By existentially becoming absorbed in the lives of others who were far worse off than she, Georgia allowed her service to completely envelop her existing personality, unconsciously, until the realization that she did not have it so bad overcame her conscious mind with subtle and unequivocal realization of a change in her existing personality and attitude.

Author William Bridges has noted that "genuine beginnings begin within us, even when they are brought to our attention by external opportunities. It is out of the formlessness of the neutral zone that new form emerges and out of the barrenness of the fallow time that new life springs."

The Buddhist religion holds that in order to realize true happiness, one must know suffering. To the Buddhists, all life is suffering, and real happiness can only be achieved in the mind within a heightened state of awareness. The four noble truths that must be recognized here to become *enlightened* are: life means suffering; the origin of suffering is attachment; the cessation of suffering is attainable; and there is a path to the cessation of suffering.

Analyzing these four noble truths tells us that we may never be able to keep permanently what we strive for due to the impermanence of all things. Thinking that the objects of attachment are transient leads us into the understanding of the meaning of impermanence and our *craving* and *clinging* desires, which make for suffering in light of not giving in to change. By allowing ourselves to cease to desire, we can break away from attachment, placing less emphasis on those entities that might not be as important to us as we once thought they were and subsequently reaching what Buddhists call Nirvana, or freedom from all worries, troubles, complexes, fabrications, and ideas.

There is a path to the end of all suffering, and apparently it is the gradual improvement of self. Becoming aware of internal change at any age is a gift in itself. To be able to change when your life is set and predictable is a notable achievement and a frightening proposition. In the end, the essence of growth is based on a person's ability to change, understand the change, and adapt to it without losing any great degree of continuity from within oneself. We can always amend the changes we encounter with more change; however, this may lead to heightened states of uncertainty and confusion.

If you are dealing with an aged individual, making changes should be slow, well thought out, and clearly communicated. Having respect for an older individual who has lived a specific type of lifestyle for many years is an essential prerequisite. It has been stated that patience is a virtue, and with elderly people patience is a necessity. One cannot rush change. Changes are based on personal attitude and our ability to either compromise in the decision-making process about change or forge ahead without regard for the consequences.

With respect to change, I am reminded of clergyman Charles Swindoll's description of attitude from an archive of his thoughts (Heart to Heart, Musings on Love, Music and Life, 2008) which reads as follows:

> *We cannot change our past ... we cannot change the fact that people will act in a certain way. We cannot change the inevitable. The only thing we can do is play on the one string that we have, and that is our attitude. I am convinced that life is 10 percent what happens to me and 90 percent how I react to it. And so it is with you ... we are in charge of our attitudes.*

Change is the lifeblood of aging. When we recognize that change is the constant in life that creates newness for us, we can set out to explore our new horizons with our inner child. A sense of wonder exists where trepidation is quelled and excitement fills the journey. Change is better explained as a process that is endless. Self-exploration is a journey that holds hands with aging and with change itself.

An elderly patient of mine always encouraged me to embrace change as an extension of breathing, for with each new breath comes a new appreciation for life and what it brings to us.

Breathing in, I calm body and soul.

Breathing out, I smile.

Living in the present moment,

I know that this is the only moment"

—*Thich Nhat Hanh, Buddhist priest*

Chapter 3

Who's on First?

MEMORY

What makes old age hard to bear is not the failing of one's faculties, mental and physical, but the burden of one's memories.

—William Somerset Maugham, English playwright

Two octogenarians were sitting on a bench together silently. Finally, Harry looked at Sidney and said, "So what's new?" Sidney looked at Harry and said in a slow, languishing tone, "Well, I have a new thirty-year-old girlfriend. We make love all night long. It's like nothing I've ever experienced. She does things to me I've only read about or seen in movies. She makes me feel thirty-five years old again. I'm in love!" he exclaimed sadly. Harry responded with, "What's to be so sad about? It sounds as if you have found the pot of gold at the end of the rainbow." Sidney replied, saying, "I have the treasure of a lifetime, but I can't remember where she lives!"

Memory loss, to be sure, can be devastating at times in our lives, wreaking havoc with everyday, mundane tasks or in remembering the finite details of how to get dressed or operate something as simple as a nail clipper.

The brain, according to the *Oxford American Desk Dictionary and Thesaurus* Second Edition, is "an organism of soft nervous tissue contained in the skull of vertebrates, responsible for being the center of sensation and of intellectual and nervous activity." I have always been fascinated by this organ system, which in itself has not one iota of sensation or sensory enervation. To think that this mass of protoplasm and associated cephalopodan, octopus-like wiring system makes all of us function the way we do.

Hardwiring our systems (referenced in research by such notable social scientists as Dr. Heinz Von Foerster) in a preordained manner, our genetics dictate how we will ultimately function physically and think mentally. However, there is never any guarantee that the way we function, once out of the womb, will be what our perception of normal will be. As we age, it is expected that some of our brain cells will not regenerate or continue to hold the same position of importance they once did for us. Simple memory loss can be found in most people as they become overtasked, overstressed and undernourished, including such things as missing meals, drinking too much alcohol, skipping a nap, and becoming tired or even dehydrated.

Lack of fluid, such as water, can wreak havoc with the mind and body. Our brains at an older age tend to play tricks on us, making us think that we don't have a need to drink water anymore. We are not as thirsty as we age for this salubrious liquid, which is approximately 90 percent of our body's makeup, as we once were. The pituitary gland, our master gland, decreases in function, thereby reducing the amount of the hormone vasopressin in the hypothalamus of the brain. This in turn causes a loss of thirst.

In states of dehydration the memory is diminished, creating a double-edged sword. Kidney disease or decreased function at an older age will also mimic similar symptoms of lack of thirst. Fooling people into dehydration, the physiology of our bodies needs to be monitored on a regular basis in order to prevent as well as treat systemic problems. Regular visits to the physician are warranted.

Memory loss, such as not being able to find the car keys, can be normal. Half the time, when I get up in the morning, I forget what appointments I have. I consider myself normal, but some people may take issue with this statement. However, as we age we do lose some cognition, and that is normal.

Recently, I had a client call me—I will call her Harriet—a nurse about fifty-five years young, who exclaimed that she could not keep up with her grandchildren anymore. When I asked her to clarify for me, she told me that she was having trouble doing simple math problems and spelling with these children. Embarrassment had set in for her, and she was reaching out for help through another woman, a friend, who referred her to me directly. One grandchild was in the third grade and the other was in the fifth grade.

It was obvious to me that was not a normal situation. I did some cognitive testing on her and found her to be compromised. This woman really had trouble doing math problems of all sorts, reading simple stories, and spelling words, as well as remembering things that happened in her life. After continued questioning, Harriet told me that she had blacked out several times over the past ten years. Fear sometimes preempts our attempts to remember important events in our histories, which may present a cause and effect scenario for cognitive problems we perceive to be happening. This was the case with Harriet, as she had a lot of trepidation about letting her husband and their respective families know that she was cognitively impaired and could not remember how to do things. Fear was the strongest barrier to recovery from this unmet need.

I referred her for a neurological workup, including a CT scan of her brain, blood tests, and further psychiatric testing. I also recommended some drug therapy for her in the form of the new drugs for dementia and Alzheimer's disease, which help with memory retention. This is a class of drugs called cholinesterase inhibitors, including the generic drugs Donepezil (Aricept), Galantamine (Reminyl), Rivastigmine (Exelon), and Tacrine (Cognex). There is also the drug Memantine HCL or Namenda, which is an NMDA-Receptor antagonist. In time there will be new memory enhancing drugs on the market that may prove better than the existing ones. New research is finding proteins that dissolve the Tau protein in the brain responsible for causing disruption of nerve impulses. These Tau proteins are produced in the brain of Alzheimer's disease patients and can be seen in an MRI or CT scan. A drug called Rember, being tested at the University of Scotland is proving to be a promising medication for dissolving the Tau proteins and reversing the effects of dementia in Alzheimer's patients. The Buck Institute for Geriatric Research in Marin County, California is also testing a new protein that dissolves the plaque that causes Alzheimer's disease.

All of these memory drugs are designed to decrease memory loss in cognitively impaired individuals. Some work better than others, and it should be up to a person's physician as to which one would be indicated for the specific situation at hand. Harriet went for testing and was subsequently placed on the drug Aricept. She also went through memory training with me, resulting in her continued improvement. I am not sure whether she ever informed her family of the fact that she had had, and continued to have, what we call TIAs or transient ischemic attacks: a series of small strokes. These events had impaired her vasculature (blood vessels), damaging parts of her brain, and subsequently causing some damage to the memory centers of her cerebral cortex. In actuality, what Harriet was experiencing was a form of vascular dementia.

When looking at specific memory loss problems, you need to play detective; that is, look at all the obvious things that can cause the problem and then delve into the more hidden list of unthinkable items that might be causing the situation at hand. This is a hit or miss effort and requires extreme diligence, persistence, and knowledge. I recommend a team approach, as two or three heads are better than one in problem-solving efforts of this nature. I recall cases where the simplest of things—"the unthinkable," I call them—were not discussed because one person thought that such a small item would or could not cause a larger problem, but we were way off base in our thinking because a minute detail was indeed the culprit.

Another example of being off-base was what occurred several years ago with my mother. She told me she had lung cancer. This was affirmed by her medical doctor and verified by three other doctors her physician had referred her to for opinions. I had asked if one simple test, an aspiration biopsy, was done to diagnosis this disease more definitively. Of course, the answer was "no" and "I trust my doctor." I was upset and demanded that my mother have this test, but she refused, not wanting to upset or insult her doctor. Needless to say, the upper right lobe of her lung was subsequently removed. Several hours afterward, a doctor, who I had not met or seen before, came into the ICU (Intensive Care Unit) to inform our family that a terrible mistake had been made. My mother did not have lung cancer; she had pneumonia! Too late to put the lung back! I did everything I could to restrain myself and not scream. If only one small test had been done, this tragedy could have been averted. Mother, the consummate optimist, was grateful that she did not have the "Big C."

As I was walking down the stair
I met a man that wasn't there.
I saw him there again today,
I wish to God he'd go away.

—Hughes Mearns, American educator and poet

We don't see what we don't see; and we don't know what we don't know.

—Dr. Heinz Von Foerster,
Personal statement to the Author

BEHIND CLOSED DOORS

Behind closed doors lie the secrets of our lives. Socrates stated that "the eyes are the windows of our souls." Just looking into someone's eyes can tell one a story about where this person is in time and space and what their emotional state might be like at the present time. This obviously takes a little experience, but usually a person with this soothsayer type of talent can determine another's state of mind.

Memory loss plays a large part in many people's lives when it comes to cloistering themselves behind closed doors. Fear, as I have alluded to, is a major player here, keeping people from acting appropriately or seeking help for their undiagnosed problems or specific challenges.

Sometimes pride gets in our way as well, or lack of knowledge about what is happening to us, and we cannot see clearly to function in a way that would keep us from harming ourselves. I had a client who I was called upon to see by the local county mental health department's senior peer counselors. This person would not come out of her home. When I knocked on her door she opened it slightly and then grabbed my arm, pulling me inside with great force all the while screaming "they're watching us!" Needless to say, I was scared and ready to fight for my life. She told me that she was being watched but could not remember by whom. She also had so many boxes, so much furniture, and other things cluttering her home, one could barely move from one place to another. She asked me to sit down in the only chair in the house not being used, which I did, and then she proceeded to tell me about the people who were watching her and listening to her.

Obviously, this person had paranoid delusions and was probably schizophrenic. She had very little memory of her personal history, whether she had any family, or even who she was. I knew that this person was way beyond the help I could give her as a peer counselor. I got out of there as soon as I could, going back to the county offices to do some research on this unfortunate woman and report her to my supervisor. This poor individual did not even go out of her home to buy food. She had some of her neighbors bring food to her. She had a son, who informed me that he was trying to have his mother committed for insanity.

I think that with some proper medication, counseling, and guidance, this woman could have had a chance to reenter a normal life. The question was whether or not someone would give her this chance. I never found out. There are many people like this who repeat this scenario and who have lost their memory banks. They are walking our streets, sitting in doorways, or are shut in their own rooms or homes, abandoned by others, having transported themselves to some other space and time. Mental illness pervades our society, yet memory loss does not necessarily indicate mental illness.

> *Look, it cannot be seen—it is beyond form.*
>
> *Listen, it cannot be heard—it is beyond sound.*
>
> *Grasp, it cannot be held—it is intangible.*
>
> *These three are indefinable:*
>
> *Therefore they are joined in one.*
>
> *From above it is not bright;*
>
> *From below it is not dark:*
>
> *An unbroken thread beyond description.*
>
> *It returns to nothingness.*
>
> *The form of the formless,*
>
> *The image of the imageless,*
>
> *It is called indefinable and beyond imagination.*
>
> *Stand before it and there is no beginning.*
>
> *Follow it and there is no end …*
>
> —*Lao Tzu, Tao Te Ching*

Certainly, form follows function. If there is no functionality in the aged or damaged person, who is lost to the doom and gloom of mental disease or memory loss, then there is not the form to follow for a normal life. Memory loss is indeed a frightening proposition for those who are touched by this insidious condition. Humor plays a part in people's fear response to memory loss as exemplified by an old joke: "The one good thing about Alzheimer's disease is that one is constantly making new friends!"

Just the thought of knowing that a close relative may be subject to this dreaded disease brings on a response that consists of denial, grief, anger, and fear. Genetic tests can provide information about propensity toward Alzheimer's disease among family members. Recent research located the gene responsible for Alzheimer's disease on gene number nineteen. There is a double pair of chromosomes there, one of which can give a predilection toward Alzheimer's and the other of which can protect against it—the yin and the yang of memory loss, so to speak. The majority of people who may be related to others who have this disease may not, by the law of averages, think that they will get it, and in that vein not avail themselves of this specific genetic testing for the disease.

To cite an example in my own family, one of my cousins discovered that the family harbored a rare gene, found in Ashkenazi Jews, that indicated a predilection toward both ovarian and breast cancers in woman and prostate and colon cancers in men. When each of my family members was notified that we should consider having a genetic test to determine whether we were victim to this the BRACA 1 and BRACA 2 genes, no one responded, at least, for about a year. The first to respond was my sister, who found that she had the gene and was subsequently faced with some difficult decisions. At age forty-eight she elected surgery to remove her ovaries and reduce her risk of contracting cancer from approximately 85 percent down to about 5 percent. I took the genetic blood test and found I did not have the specific gene. (There is a 50 percent chance that the gene is passed on to each generation.) My brother refused to take the test.

This example points to the general, approximately 66 percent, response with respect to the news a family has the gene and taking further action to see if the gene was present. I would think that my brother would invest in taking this simple test in order to know if he carried the gene, for his children's sake. One can lead a horse to water but can't make it fish.

As with some forms of memory loss that are known to have a genetic component, people can and should avail themselves of these tests in order to plan for the future. Knowing in advance that a catastrophic event may occur in one's future is half the battle in preparing for it; hence, air-raid sirens, tsunami warning systems, smoke detectors, and genetic testing, to name a few of the advanced warning systems mankind has developed to stave off misfortune.

NOW THAT YOU'VE GOT IT, WHAT DO YOU DO WITH IT?

Okay, one has discovered that his or her memory is really diminishing. Whether the progress of the loss is slow or rapid, one must first decide how to determine the extent of damage created and the damage control that one has to do to either slow the progression of the problem or stop it altogether, if possible.

Cognitive testing is in order for any kind of memory loss. The tests are simple, direct, and easy to administer by a gerontologist, social worker, psychologist, psychiatrist, neurologist, or geriatrician. Repetitive forgetfulness during the day is an indication that something is happening out of the ordinary, and it is a symptom not to take for granted. Loss of car keys, glasses or "where did I put the dog" kind of things are usually normal in the sense that sometimes we become mindless in our daily routines and do not pay much attention to where we place things. The secret for this specific challenge is to leave personal articles in the same place all the time. If one does this already and these same questions come up continuously, then there is suspicion enough to look into a memory loss problem: testing is in order.

I have a dear friend who has ADD, Attention Deficit Disorder, and he does not pay much attention to details regarding things like his car keys or reading glasses, which he constantly misplaces. This is not a case of overt memory loss but a case of attention deficit disorder and the lack of importance my friend places on these items. He frequently buys at least ten pairs of inexpensive glasses at the drugstore and leaves them all around his house, car, and office. Inevitably, I find his glasses on the couch after he visits my house or in my car if we drive somewhere. He just does not pay much attention to where he places things. The last time we went to a movie together he left his keys in his seat and had to get a pass to go back inside to retrieve them.

If my friend is upset by the fact that he has a large agenda on a specific day, then my advice to him is to write things down in order of importance so that he can remember what he needs to do next. He should also carry a small notebook, a memory book as I call it, with him to refer to on a regular basis. He will inevitably waste a lot of time looking for what he did not pay attention to, including finding the list I asked him to prepare.

One really has to laugh at this behavior rather than stress over it, since there is no other way to deal with the situation other than medication. There are various medications for ADD that can effectively slow a person down, allowing them to think more clearly and slowly about things. As I have told my students in the past, "We think four times faster than we can hear, so if you finish the lecture I am giving before I do, then you are free to leave."

Because our minds are always going a mile a minute, we must find ways to slow down and concentrate on what we are dealing with in the moment, not necessarily what we are thinking about for the immediate future. There are also drugs to enhance memory, as I have discussed earlier in this book. These can help the mind in assimilating information better and helping messages become understood a lot easier and faster so that the recipient remembers them instead of letting them just go by unconsciously.

Severe memory loss can be discerned as either short-term or long-term memory loss. Usually, short-term memory loss is acute and indicates a possible CVA, cerebral vascular accident, or TIA, transient ischemic attack, both of which are strokes due to vascular blood clots in the brain. The cause of these problems, such as blood clots, can be pinpointed to clots that have been created in other parts of the body, that float free and travel from these other areas of the body, due to injury or as a result of recent surgery or events that occur naturally, or they may also be nothing more than fat globules displaced from a surgical site traveling to an area that will cause harm. Hardening of the arteries, or atherosclerosis as it has been labeled, can lead to a slow deterioration of the memory banks and significant long-term memory loss. Usually, vascular dementia is related to this kind of situation.

I once had a client who had suffered several brain aneurysms, whereby the main artery in the brain ruptured causing bleeding within the brain itself and subsequent damage to the client and her ability to function properly. This person's speech center was affected by the damage as well as her ability to walk or move parts of her body. She had two of these events within a short period of time with subsequent surgical intervention. One of the surgeries may have led to a stroke, as well, causing memory loss along with everything else that had occurred.

I was called in to do an assessment of the client and her caregivers, who were suspected of abusing the client emotionally and financially. It is interesting to note at this juncture that care should be taken in having caregivers help with physically and cognitively impaired individuals when no family or case manager is present to monitor their behavior and make sure they are trained for this type of patient with these specific problems. Primarily due to the fact that this client was cognitively impaired, the caregivers used certain tactics to extract money from the client through guilt-provoking behavior as well as abusing her emotionally.

The client could not remember what she had relinquished to her caregivers but did remember that she had been forced into giving them money and that she argued with them. The client had a ballistic temper due to her injury and created much havoc amongst her caregivers and others who visited her from time to time. Having a memory deficit for someone like this woman was essentially to her detriment. She could not really remember all the details about things that happened to her, but she knew that things happened that she did not like.

Making the best out of a bad situation is an important act under dire circumstances. This is a time where family or good friends should be involved in the improvement and acceptance phase of memory loss, leading to emotional healing. Sometimes things are more painful for those of us who may not be affected mentally but who are mere bystanders trying to help our loved ones in ways that we are uncertain about and without knowledge to do so. This can be considered most frustrating. When children of parents who are gradually losing their memory get involved, there can be much confusion, differences of opinions, and verbal fighting. Everyone seems to know what he or she thinks is best for the parent, but in reality, the parent or parents should have dictated their desires for care long before any demise. Unfortunately, this is not always the case and leads to family crisis and consternation.

Some time ago, I received a call from a woman who was of Latin extraction. She complained that her eighty-six-year-old mother was not only losing her memory but also was a closet drinker. My client was upset because her mother was left alone all day to fend for herself, while her sister, with whom she stayed, worked all day. None of her other brothers or sisters did anything to share the burden of helping the mother. My client was the youngest sister of the family. She was a nurse, meticulous, had a wonderful family of her own, and was most dedicated to taking care of her family, including her mother, for whom she felt responsible.

I asked my client to call a family meeting so that we could all talk together. The day of the intended meeting, I showed up at my client's home to find at least ten brothers and sisters present sitting around an enormous table in the dining room, mimicking some corporate board meeting for General Motors. I was in shock! Half the siblings spoke English, and the other half spoke Spanish. This was going to be like hitting a wall, I thought. Lots of fun …

A time to talk,

A time to listen,

A time to think,

Listen and watch what's at stake.

A time to give in,

A time to wait,

A time to invest,

A whole family to make.

A cohesive group,

An unending loop,

A family that dares,

A family that cares.

A circus of acts that make one smile,

A menagerie of thoughts lasting a while.

——*Eric Zane Shapira, "The Meeting"*

I proceeded to ask each sibling to tell the others present what he or she did to help dear old mom, when he or she performed this act of benevolence, how often, and what perceptions each had regarding the care mom was presently receiving on a daily basis. I wanted to see if my clients' perceptions or chief complaints were justified and if everyone was on the same page. As it turned out, the left hand did not know what the right hand was doing.

This situation seemed like a fourteen-ring circus: different acts, different perceptions, and a total lack of focus on the issue at hand—mom. Many of the brothers, I think about five of them, were in agreement with the idea of allowing mom to have a nip of alcohol now and then. However, these people didn't know that their mother was unsupervised and they were unaware that mom hit the bottle hard nightly, sometimes drinking until she fell flat on her face, dead drunk. This was both unacceptable and dangerous due to the mother's fragility, her age, and the high risk of hip fracture, which at her age would be devastating and life threatening. Just the fact that the brothers even thought the way they did was infuriating to the sisters, and the result was a rift among them all.

All in all, the meeting took about two hours and was conducted in both English and Spanish to the satisfaction of the audience. I thought I would try something new, since there was so much dissention among the family at this point. I formed a mock corporation with the family, each becoming a stakeholder in the corporation. What was the business of this corporation, you ask? The mother, of course. Each stakeholder agreed to agree and agreed to disagree. Each person agreed to take on an active role in their mother's care. Some of the children could only agree to call her daily on the telephone rather than spend the time to go see her, while others agreed to spend time with her, bringing their respective families to be with her at least once per week. Mom was okay with all of these commitments.

The business flourished for several years and then one day, out of the blue, I received a call from my original client, the youngest sister, who asked me to facilitate another corporate meeting with her siblings. Upon invitation, about half of the siblings showed up for the meeting. Several of the ones who were present had not lived up to their end of the bargain. This time the mother was invited to attend the meeting, a new twist. Mom had moved into my client's home, where a new room and bath had been added since our last meeting there. The client was most happy to have her mother living with her. My client had arranged for care for her mother during the week at my suggestion and treated the alcohol problem by giving Mom a prescription dose (one diluted glass of wine) at bedtime as a sedative to help her sleep. During the day, mother went to the local senior center and traded off with the adult day-health center, where she received meals and therapy and socialization. Mom was picked up by bus at about nine in the morning and returned about five in the afternoon, just in time to meet her daughter returning from work. My client wished her siblings would give her some respite on the weekends. That was arranged during our second corporate meeting. So far, so good.

For the memory impaired person, it is important to have consistency in care along with constant mental stimulation. It is not enough to place Mom in front of the TV and let her stare at it for hours on end, not knowing if she is getting anything of value out of it or even understanding what she may be watching. Sending her to the senior center and adult day-health center allowed Momma maximum mental stimulation, ambulation, and socialization. Returning her each day to her daughter's house, being with family, grandchildren and the like, helped give Momma the consistency, continuity and familiarity that she needed to stabilize her memory loss.

It is interesting to note that families in crisis tend to display desperate behavior, which in turn can cause a great stir in family dynamics with resultant hysteria emanating from "I don't know what to do with mom or dad!" It takes a search for a gerontologist who can help with family mediation on aging issues to mitigate hysteria and unreasonableness within the family. Individuals may act out on behalf of his or her parents, actually making things worse in the long run.

Having confused and angry children only exacerbates the confusion, frustration, and lost feelings of the parent or parents in question, who themselves are in crisis. Memory loss, with its frustration, causes a person to become upset, irritable, and unsure about everything that presents itself. The one who is affected by such damage experiences a continuous bombardment of alien messages, signs, symptoms, and incomprehensible barbs. Dodging such barbs is almost impossible for the memory-impaired person who cannot interpret the meaning of questions, let alone recognize faces of the loved ones in his or her life.

It is sad to think that the mind can be bathed in a sea of ignorance blinding even the most astute eye from the natural light of day. Memory loss equates to change, and change subsequently creates dissonance and inadequacies in the memory-impaired individual who cannot process this change. Changes due to memory loss require shifting of and flexibility in family dynamics and roles. People will ultimately have better positive mental health and understanding around these sometimes subtle differences if they can adapt, yet keep something of their own creativity. This in turn will promote better acceptance and attitude. Total loss meets with resistance and especially denial for all parties concerned. So, we need to help each other adapt to the changes and differences brought upon us or our loved ones by experiencing memory loss and confusion.

> *I am alone,*
>
> *With the stillness of my thoughts;*
>
> *Seeking tenderness from anyone who will give it…*
>
> *I ache, in the stillness of the night;*
>
> *Who dares to comfort me? Who wishes to share their love?*
>
> *I do not think of feelings directly,*
>
> *I only remember them in glimmering flashes;*
>
> *The love, the touch, the tenderness I once had…*
>
> —Eric Zane Shapira, "I Am Alone"

And in turn one who is alone with his or her own thoughts, bathed in obscurity, becomes the "silent sufferer" needing to be understood, nurtured, loved, and eventually reborn. Without the qualities of understanding, patience, nurturing, caring, flexibility, and information about the memory loss condition, there will be no peace between caregiver and those affected by this catastrophic condition.

> *Suffering in silence, longing…*
>
> *Longing for a tuned-in ear;*
>
> *Longing for a place without fear;*
>
> *The forgotten gesture, the additional act.*
>
> —Eric Zane Shapira, "The Silent Sufferer"

WHAT ABOUT THE CAREGIVER?

Who is chosen as a caregiver is an important facet of caring for a person with memory loss or anyone who is medically compromised or disabled in some way. One must think long and hard about a specific type of caregiver or caregiver service. Today, we are inundated with caregiver services. These are listed as home-health agencies, caregiver agencies, affordable living agencies and assisted-living facilities.

> ***Helpful Hint:*** You might look for certified home-health aides in the want ads of the local newspaper, call the local senior center for referrals for caregivers who are known to the agency, or call the county department of aging and adult services, which may maintain a list of agencies and independent companies that provide care.

It is difficult, to say the least, to find someone to take care of a loved one, especially when you are not sure what you are looking for with respect to skills and empathy. Recently, I had a young woman wanting a caregiver qualified as an RN (Registered Nurse) for her mother who needed medical care along with caregiving in general. This is a tall order and a costly one. I suggest that people first sit down with their loved one, and if they are able, ask what kind of person the patient would like to have with them daily to spend time with them and care for them. I have had people in a variety of circumstances request a myriad of different kinds of people. There were those who did not want a foreigner.

That's unfortunate, because foreign caregivers are often excellent, patient- devoted, kind, and very experienced. Many of them come with nursing and medical backgrounds from their countries but are unable, for one reason or another, to become licensed here. The majority of foreign caregivers in the United States are from Latin American, Philippine, Samoan, Fijian, and Indian cultures. Very few caregivers in general are Caucasian, white Euro-Americans, in origin.

There are caregivers who are bonded; caregivers who are certified; caregivers who are in the United States illegally, yet have advanced medical degrees; caregivers who have identification cards but no Social Security card; and any number of combinations. Many caregivers want room and board in their work environment. Most want to be paid in cash.

I had a client who had three caregivers providing care twenty-four hours a day and seven days a week. Each was paid every two weeks by a conservator, and each received a bonus now and then for their work. Each one received a cash birthday gift as well, but none of them were covered for worker's comp insurance, or liability, or medical insurance for themselves or family members. I told the conservator that she was running a business because the three caregivers had been procured from an agency for a fee but were not paid by the agency directly, which made them employees of the conservatorship. The conservatorship was liable for all the expenses of these caregivers and should have incorporated as a business or hired these people under a trust agreement of some sort. The conservator insisted these people were all independent contractors. It is best to think about consulting an attorney to make a ruling on the type of business relationship you decide to have before hiring one or more caregivers. These are things you must think about before hiring independent people.

There was another client of mine who wanted me to go to see her mother some six hundred miles from my office and do an assessment of her situation. I was more than happy to do so, but the client preempted me by going to see her mother by herself when an emergency occurred.

First of all, the caregiver, after working for the mother for over ten years, out of the blue, demanded a contract and a salary of eighty thousand dollars a year with benefits! She had been paid much less than this figure, with no benefits prior to the demand. She told the daughter that if her new demands were not met, she would then demand overtime pay for the past ten years. At this point, the daughter did an investigation, after consulting with me, and found that the caregiver and the caregiver's daughter, who substituted for her mom on the weekends, had been stealing funds from my client's mother, who suffered from memory loss, for over nine years.

What an awakening! Here was the scam: Whenever the caregiver needed to go shopping, the mother would give her a blank check. The caregivers would make the check out for much more than the sum of their purchases and keep the difference. This was discovered after some days of hard work comparing the checks to the receipts for purchases and thoroughly investigating all the financials of the mother. The caregivers were subsequently arrested and sent off to jail.

> ***Helpful Hint:*** It is important to remember to keep all receipts and place them in a file under day, date, and time, as well as who made the purchase and who gave the authorization to make the purchase.

Subsequently, my client contracted with an agency, which was bonded, and hired two caregivers part-time to cover a full range of time with her mother. Each caregiver was salaried by the agency, insured, and paid regular employee benefits, as they should be.

I cite these examples because most people do not even think about the ramifications of hiring caregivers for a loved one, other than the overall cost to them and how they will begin to pay for someone like this. Other details are sometimes skipped over, and this is what gets people into trouble. Many times I am asked to come into a household and screen the caregivers for improprieties or efficiency. In List One (below), I have assembled a list of what to look for in a caregiver, should you desire to hire one, either independently or through an agency. Please note that you might still wish to overlook some of the details to save on costs, or you may not find someone with all the characteristics that you are looking for and settle on something other than what you originally desired, but in the long run, this may come back to bite you where it hurts—your pocketbook—as well as in your peace of mind.

What to Look for in a Caregiver

Here is a list of questions to ask when looking for a caregiver. The list is by no means comprehensive, but it covers the most important considerations.

1. Is the caregiver a certified Home Health Aide? Will the cost be different if they are?
2. Is the caregiver trained, or better yet certified, in CPR?
3. Does the agency pay his or her salary?
4. Does the caregiver have liability and worker's compensation insurance coverage?
5. Does the caregiver have medical benefits?
6. What are the expectations of the agency and the caregiver regarding work hours and time off? Can the caregiver adhere to the family's schedule??
7. How long has the caregiver been at this job and employed by this particular agency?
8. Has the caregiver had a background check? Credit check?
9. Does the caregiver have a valid driver's license and does he or she own a car?

10. Can the caregiver drive the patient to appointments and run errands as needed?
11. Does the caregiver speak, read, and understand English? What is the caregiver's native language?
12. Will the caregiver's health or physical condition affect performance? Are they able to lift at least 50-100 pounds?
13. Does the caregiver have any physical health problems?
14. Has the caregiver had emergency first-aid training?
15. What kind of personal skills does the caregiver have (cooking and personal attendance to activities of daily living)?
16. What kind of communication style does the caregiver have (empathic vs. sympathetic)?
17. How good is the caregiver's ability to learn new information?
18. What is the demeanor and personal hygiene of the caregiver?
19. How well does the caregiver take directions?
20. What special skills and attributes does the caregiver have?
21. Is the caregiver flexible?
22. Does the caregiver have references? May we contact them?
23. Does the caregiver have any special considerations (likes and dislikes, disabilities, allergy to pets, for example)?
24. Does the caregiver have any licenses or certifications?
25. Does the caregiver work well with others?
26. Would the caregiver be amenable to taking a personality test (MMPI, Disc Analysis, Taylor-Johnson Temperament Analysis, or another type of personality trait test)?
27. What is the basic salary requirement of the caregiver, and do they expect overtime pay?
28. What kind of preferences or expectations does the caregiver have with respect to a client?

29. Will the caregiver agree in advance on an annual cost-of-living raise?
30. Does the caregiver have family nearby? Elsewhere in the U.S.?
31. How long does the caregiver expect to stay in the United States?

If you hire from an agency make sure the agency is bonded and insured. Make sure the agency has contingency plans in case the hired caregiver does not show up. Make sure the agency is a member of the Better Business Bureau and/or the local Chamber of Commerce. This way if something negative happens to you, there may be recourse through arbitration or mediation with these organizations. Make sure to get some references from people who have used the agency you are looking at, and be sure to compare various agencies in the area for consistency and services that are offered.

MEMORY LOSS WITH AGING: WHAT'S NORMAL, WHAT'S NOT

Have you found yourself saying "What?" very often? Do you wonder if your hearing is going or you just can't remember what was said just a few seconds ago? You know that you left the car keys on the dresser where you always leave them but they are not there! Gosh darn it all ... where did I put them? Or even worse, you come out of the market into that big parking lot where you left your car and it looks like the Bermuda Triangle: "Where is my car?" you think to yourself.

Well, you are not losing your mind, you're just being normal for the most part. In today's generation, we find ourselves in a fast-food, fast-paced, "do it now" society. We tend to clutter our brains with so many things at one time it is no wonder we can't even remember who we are or where we are supposed to be going. When you are in your twenties, you begin to lose brain cells a few at a time. Your body starts to make less of the chemicals your brain cells need to work. The older you are the more of these changes can affect your memory.

Aging may affect your memory by changing the way the brain stores information and by making it harder to recall stored information. Usually, your short-term and remote memories are not affected by aging. But your recent memory may be affected within an hour of observing or learning something or an action you took within that hour. The examples I just mentioned, or even forgetting names of people you may have met recently, are normal changes. Most of these little nuisances are just the normal brain trying to prioritize, sort, store, and retrieve this information. Frequent memory lapses tend to be noticeable because they interfere with normal living. Let's look at a brain and your memory.

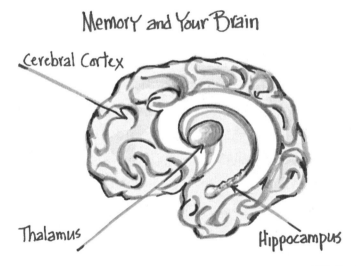

© E. Shapira 2009

The cerebral cortex is where we have formed memories and stored them. The thalamus is considered to have a role in the formation of new memories partly through the relationship with the hippocampus. Both of these areas are important for mental alertness. The hippocampus itself is believed to be critical in the formation of new memories. Direct injury to any of these areas can impair your ability to retrieve or store memory.

The amygdala is a part of the brain that is one of the hottest topics of neuro-research today. It is an area deep in the brain that connects one's emotions to the memories stored in the hippocampus. Being able to find joy in memory loss may be tied into a memory impaired individual's ability to retrieve information from the amygdala, translated by the hippocampus, and brought forth to the mind's eye for a reaction from within the person. Hence, retrieving a lost memory will inevitably make a memory impaired person happy realizing that they can now remember something they had difficulty understanding. This may happen in bits and pieces, still creating frustration at the same time. My mother-in-law, who had a small stroke, can see the word she wants to use but sometimes can't get a hold of it in her mind to say it. The times she is able to grasp the word and "spit it out" makes her quite happy and content.

Causes of Memory Loss

Memory loss can also be caused by the following:

1. Normal aging. Aging may make it more difficult to have proper recall.
2. Medications, such as sleeping pills, over-the-counter antihistamines, antianxiety pills, antidepressants, medication for schizophrenia, and pain medications, especially after a surgery.
3. Alcohol and illicit drug use. Heavy alcohol use depletes Vitamin B1 (Thiamine), which can harm memory. Marijuana and heavier drug use block out memory.

4. General stress. Stress particularly due to emotional trauma can cause memory loss. In rare cases, amnesia can result. Post Traumatic Stress Disorder (PTSD) is a phenomenon that suppresses memories that are too terrible in one's mind to remember. The victim may find these memories or fleeting glimpses of them sneaking out at times, creating panic attacks, crying, or depression. These memories may be triggered by totally unrelated instances that are related in the person's unconscious, triggering a replay of the original trauma and provoking an aberrant response. This type of disorder needs psychological treatment. Various modalities in treatment have been discovered, such as EMDR, a rapid eye movement technique that brings forth the trauma, to try and heal the trauma of these PTSD patients and facial tapping techniques as well. Brain spotting, a new technique is on the rise for treating trauma and memory problems.
5. Depression is common in aging and can cause a lack of attention and focus on memory.
6. Head injury.
7. Systemic diseases and Infections. HIV, TB, syphilis, herpes, and other infections of the lining of the brain may cause memory loss.
8. Thyroid dysfunction. An underactive or overactive thyroid can interfere with memory.
9. Nutritional deficiencies. Vitamin B1 and B12 deficiency can affect memory.
10. Mild cognitive impairment. This is a memory deficit beyond what is expected for normal aging.
11. Dementia. A term used for increasing impairment of memory and other aspects of thinking. There are many causes, such

as stroke or aneurysm. Alzheimer's disease is an increasingly common form of dementia with a progressive loss of brain cells.

Helpful Hint: Things to do if you notice memory failure:

- Keep lists and prioritize them by importance.
- Follow a routine.
- Make associations (connect things in your mind), such as using landmarks to help you find places; relate peoples names to a feature they may have.
- Keep a detailed calendar.
- Put important items such as keys in the same place every time.
- Repeat names when you meet new people and write them down in a little memory book you carry with you.
- Keep a journal of daily activity. Be sure to paste business cards you get from people next to an entry in the journal of their names and note the circumstances under which you met.
- Do things to keep your mind active and body busy.
- Run through the ABCs in your head to help you think of words you are having trouble remembering. "Hearing" the first letter of a word may jog your memory.
- Keep a running journal and write your thoughts down, and keep a second file on your computer.
- Use a tape recorder or MP3 player to record where you put things and your thoughts during the day. You can then copy them to your journal, your memory book, or your computer. This way, by repetition, you can help your brain remember things better.

Now where did I put my glasses? Okay, right at the end of my nose. I have learned much from my elders whose memories are diminishing. The first thing is to laugh at yourself when you make a blunder due to memory loss. The second is not to get too frustrated during the process of trying to remember what it is you forgot. Recovering your memory is challenging, to say the least, and hard work. You can make it fun, interesting, and a learning-relearning experience. Remember, attitude is everything.

Chapter 4

An Apple a Day

AGING AND CHRONIC DISEASE

Go placidly amid the noise and the haste,
And remember what peace there may be in silence.
As far as possible, without surrender,
Be on good terms with all persons.
You are a child of the universe,
No less than the trees and the stars.

—Max Ehrmann, Desiderata (excerpt)

In the beginning, there was silence, peace, and tranquility, once the firmament subsided. When man arrived on the scene in a pristine state, only then did torment, angst, stress, and disease begin to exist, disrupting the peace that pervaded the universe, or so we envision. Pestilence and disease have affected mankind from time immemorial. The human race has done its best to erase the blights that have descended upon it—ever seeking truth, balance, and longevity, but the unexpected keeps happening. Microbes may be smarter than humans.

Disease of all kinds continues, as do man's efforts to try to stop it from annihilating all living things.

Is it illusion or is it blindness that prevents man from ultimate health and discovering the Fountain of Youth? I don't think anyone really knows, but it sure would be nice to find utopia. In the later years of my practice, I noticed that more and more of my patients had had plastic surgery, sometimes repeatedly. Beauty in the form of staving off aging and disease was in the forefront of each and every one who drank from the "well," referencing the Fountain of Youth idea. Is it a sign of the times? I think so. Is this how people learn to make peace with the aging process? Possibly, but I believe there is more to it than this move to be more beautiful and younger looking through plastic surgery.

In a study that I conducted with dental students more than twenty-five years ago in a local San Francisco skilled nursing facility, as part of a school course that I developed to teach diagnosis and treatment planning, findings from head and neck exams suggested that approximately 8 percent of those ambulatory patients examined had medical problems that went undiagnosed by a physician. Could this be in our perfect society? The simple answer is yes. Many people do not understand disease or know its symptoms. And, unfortunately, many people get lost in the system in nursing homes and facilities, like this one surveyed, only to find that regular care by a physician means being seen maybe once a year. And "being seen" means just that, being seen but not thoroughly examined.

Disease comes in many forms and sizes and can be most insidious at times, creating problems without our knowing about it. For example, my sister-in-law went in for a routine hernia repair several years ago. In the process of a laparoscopic procedure (one using several small incision holes in the belly and a camera to guide the instruments) a non-painful and unknown cancerous tumor was found on her ovary. If she had not gone in for the hernia repair, she might have been found dead one morning without anyone knowing why. Disease knows no age limits, boundaries, or barriers. It is what it is: a timeless bandit that can steal one's will and sap's one's strength, energy, and resources.

Lack of money is a factor that may add to our ability to remain ignorant in the face of personal adversity. Without resources, many people just wait for their ills to subside or end up facing death sooner than expected. I know from experience that as incomes decline, so does people's ability to seek out healthcare; hence, personal health diminishes. Without knowing the cause or symptoms of a disease that plagues them, people may often go about their daily routine not cognizant that he or she may have a communicable disease, a disease that is chronic or self-limiting.

The famous humorist, Will Rogers, once said that "Everybody is ignorant, only on different subjects." I would have to say this may be true in general, but disease is different. Disease is something that older people know something about because of personal experience; however, many people do not understand the dynamic it creates especially during the aging process. Depending upon the specific disease or malady, physical debilitation or mental deterioration can limit the ability to understand the situation or take steps to correct it. On the other hand, many people rely on their personal physician to tell them what they have and how to get rid of it. Treatment may be simple, involved or non-existent. The case with my mother's needing a needle biopsy, in my opinion, fell on deaf ears, because my mom trusted her doctor too much.

I am reminded of the old joke about a man who died and went to heaven. There he is greeted by St. Peter who talks to him for a while and then asks him if he is hungry and of course, after a long trip the man replies, "I'm famished." They go to heaven's cafeteria where there is a long line of angels waiting to get their trays all filled with abundant heavenly food. Suddenly, out of the blue, appears a guy in a green scrub suit, an obvious health professional. He rushes around, grabs a tray and utensils and then cuts in line in front of everyone else to get his food and then rushes off. With that, the new man in heaven spouts off, "Who was that cutting in line like that? I thought here in heaven everything was fair and equal." St. Peter looks at him and calmly says, "Oh, that was God, He thinks he's a doctor!" Need I say more?

When one looks at disease, chronic versus acute, systemic versus localized, and treatable versus nontreatable types, there needs to be a differentiation of what that disease is in order to cope with and subsequently treat the problem at hand. Age plays a part in all of these categories because age brings with it specific psychological and physiologic changes in one's ability to heal, cope, adapt, and fight diseases of all sorts.

Chronic disease brings on a long siege of care and treatment as well as a variety of symptoms which can be sometimes most compromising. Acute situations require immediate action and treatment to stop any long-term damage. Systemic disease is illness that affects the entire body, including the organ systems and general function of the body. Localized disease is usually manageable and curable within a short amount of time and is generally easier to treat in the long run. Diseases that are not treatable are, for the most part, life threatening and ultimately fatal. Some may become chronic in nature and last for many years, such as emphysema. This lung disease may be ultimately fatal but could last twenty years before the patient's demise.

It is difficult to predict how long someone will live when encumbered by any disease. Periodontal disease, or gum disease, is a silent, long-standing disease of the gum tissue and supporting structures of the teeth. It is not life threatening in itself but can lead to and is connected to cardiovascular disease and other systemic diseases like diabetes, which can be life threatening. The miracles of modern medicine have allowed mankind to extend life spans into the nineties and beyond, whereas around the year 1900, the average age at death was around forty-seven. The old piano player, Eubie Blake, once said, when he was one hundred years old, "If I had known I was going to live this long, I would have taken better care of myself!" So true, so true!

We tend to take a lot of things for granted as humans, one of them being our health. We often believe we are indestructible and impervious to having bad things happen to us, which is positive thinking but the wrong deduction. We, as fallible humans, need to learn to protect ourselves by eating the correct foods, exercising regularly, staying in the mainstream by being social, and stimulating our minds to keep our memories sharp and our brains clear of clutter. No one can do it for us and we will never leave our footsteps in the sands of time by sitting on our backsides.

A balanced lifestyle is recommended for longevity. The Surgeon General of the United States constantly revamps the requirements for exercise and issues warnings for discontinuing smoking because being addicted to habits of this kind is one of the hazards preventing us from living a healthy and disease-free life. President Obama just initiated an antismoking bill in Congress, a first step towards eliminating a focus of disease in our country regarding the use of tobacco. There are many bad habits in our culture and smoking, poor diet, drinking, and taking illicit drugs are but a few that will shorten our lifespan, having been statistically proven lethal over time.

If You Can Imagine It, You Can Do It

Creativity is one aspect of our lives that has not been looked at much with respect to old age; however, it has been said that creative ability has a tendency to influence longevity. I met a woman almost thirty years ago who was seventy-five years young. She was both a poet and an artist, a painter to be exact. Her name was Greer and she was most kind, gentle, pure of heart, and encouraging as well as prolific with her painting and writing of Haiku poetry. Greer lived to be about ninety years old; still writing, still painting, still practicing meditation and always the consummate vegetarian in her diet regimen. Her life was full and there was an aura about her that led one to believe that she was most accepting of her age, no matter what it was, and of life in general.

Greer was the consummate optimist when it came to encouragement. No matter what ailed her, she was grateful for what she had, rather than complaining about what was lost to her as life passed her by. She was happy to be alive and loved doing what she did. I can never remember a time that she did not prompt me to continue my own writing and constantly encouraged my ability to sculpt. Her love was unconditional, unprovoked, and always free to be handed out in gaping spoonfuls if one needed some medicine to pick them up out of the doldrums. I think her ability to be creative spilled into all aspects of her life and to everyone with whom she came into contact in her lifetime. It was infectious to a fault.

I know that I will never forget her. I also know that Greer suffered for many years from the "Big C." She never let on that she was afflicted or fighting this dreaded, pending doom, nor did she complain at all. Some days were more difficult for her than others with respect to her daily routine of painting, writing, or even getting out of bed to get dressed, but she never gave up or stopped until her light diminished. I also think that Greer's creativity kept her memory intact as much as possible. She was bright, lucid, and loquacious right up to her final moments.

Norman Cousins has stated that he learned that a highly developed purpose in life and the will to live are among the prime raw materials of human existence. Cousins met Pablo Casals, the great musician known principally for playing the cello, when he was in his eighties and continued the relationship all through Casals's nineties. Cousins was convinced that in spite of Casals's emphysema and rheumatoid arthritis, the artist continued to play the piano (a secondary instrument for him) daily to strengthen his ailing body, crippled hands and failing spirit. After playing for an hour before breakfast, Casals seemed to walk better and stand taller, and enjoyed a better appetite because of his efforts to stimulate his creative juices and loosen the joints in his hands, according to Cousins. I am sure that this regimen also allowed Casals a greater flexibility and ability to play his beloved cello.

> *You, O Fortitude,*
>
> *Purveyor of inner will and strength*
>
> *Conquering the Ages;*
>
> *Overcoming fear, pain, hurt and sorrow,*
>
> *Bringing peace to the weary*
>
> *And joy to the downtrodden sufferer.*
>
> *You, O Fortitude,*
>
> *Sage for all Ages;*
>
> *Mentor to those*
>
> *Who look deep within themselves*
>
> *To find refuge.*
>
> —Eric Zane Shapira, "O Fortitude"

At the time of this writing, Jo, my mother-in-law, at the age of ninety-three, is still an avid painter, designer, and entrepreneur. I believe that her willingness to continue promoting her creative side keeps her active, clearheaded, healthy, full of life and interesting. Her activities allow her to continue a lifestyle that she has adapted to by swimming daily for an hour or so, walking and working in her garden, taking daily afternoon naps, painting when the mood strikes her and to the extreme, buying houses and fixing them up through redesign with extensive remodeling. All of these activities give her much joy and satisfaction. She certainly is an example for all of us, young and old, who need a role model in life.

About five years ago, Jo suffered a small stroke after her husband of over sixty years passed away. I am convinced that the sudden loss and abandonment by her partner created such stress and loneliness for Jo that her blood pressure got the best of her resulting in a TIA, (transient ischemic attack). This small stroke debilitated her somewhat with respect to her memory and her ability to say words that she could visualize but not articulate. This she found most frustrating. Jo's innate stubbornness kept her from acknowledging that she needed a speech therapist as well as a grief counselor at first, but after agreeing to follow my suggestions, the local hospice was able to send in a counselor on a regular basis to help Jo overcome some of her debilities.

I was talking with Jo one day and started, off the cuff, speaking Spanish to her, just for the heck of it, knowing that she had studied this language for years. To my surprise, Jo spoke back to me in a logical and meaningful manner. Yes, it was in correct Spanish and it flowed easily from her lips. I discovered that even though her primary speech center in the cerebral cortex may have been damaged to the extent of damaging her native English language speaking center, her secondary speech center went undamaged allowing her to continue speaking very well in Spanish. We continue to converse in Spanish often, but also I push the envelope with my mother-in-law by forcing Jo to speak to me in English as well, which remains more difficult for her most of the time.

The brain is a very interesting computer of sorts. Research over the past five years has proven the brain is able to heal itself if stimulated specifically where damage has been isolated due to neurological deficit and stroke. Neurological physical therapy using electronic feedback, stimulation and repetition have helped neurologically impaired individuals regain use of lost functions. More recent research has shown that direct intervention into the damaged parts of brains can be coupled with computers so that stroke and accident victims can just think something and the computer will activate their body parts or even a wheelchair to respond. It is truly remarkable.

Several years ago, I had the pleasure of going to Chile for a humanitarian visit and met someone whose mother also had suffered a stroke, which damaged her major speech center. The eighty-plus-year-old woman could not speak her native tongue, Spanish, well enough to be understood clearly. I suggested to this woman's daughter that she encourage her mother to try to speak in English with her, this being her mother's secondary language. And, true to form, the daughter was able to converse quite easily in English with her mother, just as I had been able to speak with my mother-in-law in Spanish. What an amazing discovery! Maybe this finding will ultimately help others who have had similar experiences with parents who have been encumbered by a stroke resulting in posttraumatic stress to the speech center of the brain, compromising his or her ability to talk. The brain will heal itself to some extent, often improving after as much as a year or more. Forcing oneself to speak when speech is compromised or exercise when a certain limb is not responsive due to a stroke will inevitably bring back some of the normal function. It is critical to try and not give up.

Dr. Eric Z. Shapira, DDS, MA, MHA

DEMENTIA AND ALZHEIMER'S DISEASE

I was going to leave this section completely blank but decided that I would err on the side of not being funny with this heading, as many people may find my humor an affront to their personal experience with these diseases.

Dementia is not fun by any means and strikes many people in our country. The most common type of dementia is seen in the elderly. This affects more than four million Americans today and is a growing concern. Alzheimer's disease, on the other hand, is a progressive neurological disorder with loss of short-term memory as a prominent first sign. This disease results in: memory loss, personality change, global cognitive dysfunction, and functional impairments.

Dementia has been defined by distinct memory impairment and one or more of the following: aphasia (language problems); apraxia (simple activity challenges, e.g., buttoning); agnosis (visual recognizing problems) and executive dysfunction (e.g., driving a car). Dementia, as I have mentioned before, can be brought about by stroke or cerebral vascular accidents, TIAs, or hardening of the arteries, which occurs over time.

My father had a transient case of dementia after cardiac surgery. Sometimes the anesthesia that is delivered over a long surgery can cause memory lapse and functional difficulty after the surgery. This is usually self limiting, and normal function resumes in time. If the normal functions do not come back then, dementia sets in as a disease caused by the surgery itself and may continue for a long time thereafter.

Alzheimer's disease can be definitively diagnosed by performing a biopsy of brain tissue, having an MRI or CAT scan to determine the extent of protein plaque formation in the cortex of the brain, and now a genetic test to determine if gene nineteen appears to have the significant chromosomes responsible for the disease. The verdict is still out on specific cures for these problems, but extensive research is being conducted in many countries to try to reverse the symptoms of these disease states. Several recent research studies have shown promise with an enzyme that dissolves the protein plaques that create memory loss and brain dysfunction.

I remember a specific situation during my internship when I was examining an Alzheimer's patient in a skilled-nursing facility. While I was talking with him, a woman approached and asked me to do the same to her, at the same time lifting her blouse, exposing her breasts to me, while continuing to chat and smile as if the only thing she was doing was talking to me. I tried to act normal but this sort of thing took me by surprise, and I did everything I could to not crack a smile. The loss of inhibitions is much greater in this disease state than with drinking alcohol and getting drunk or with dementia in general. At times you can't help but laugh at the absurdities, but at the same time you feel compassion, and consider the source of the absurdity, the location it is occurring in and the situation at hand.

I suppose if this woman had been my relative, I might have been prone to reprimand her or make a case for her to stop the behavior. But one cannot be rational with an irrational person or a person who in this case probably had no idea that what she was doing was wrong. My guess is she had no idea what she was doing at all. I just acted like nothing was happening out of the ordinary and told her that as soon as I was finished with her neighbor I would stop by her "house" (a term used to refer to her room in the facility) to talk with her. She was very happy with this and asked if I knew where she lived, which I said I did. And so be it, she put her blouse down and went her way like nothing unusual had happened.

Assessments for this type of problem are complicated and require two to three hours at the least. They include cognitive testing, functional testing, and monitoring the capacity for the person in question to do certain functions like driving or dressing, doing taxes, and making decisions about medical care and related finances. This kind of testing coupled with MRI and CAT scan testing of the brain and possibly a genetic blood test are necessary to be definitive about Alzheimer's disease.

MILD COGNITIVE IMPAIRMENT

Memory loss has been associated with the aging process for many years now. Over the last few years, the medical profession has changed how it views the memory loss problems of elders and in light of the so-called "senior moments" comments, a category of disease indicative of a memory deficit has developed to categorize mild cognitive memory loss or impairment. For the most part, MCI (mild cognitive impairment) is considered not normal and a medical debility with respect to the probability that it will evolve into a more advanced state of dementia, with significant changes in permanent memory. MCI may be a precursor to dementia and Alzheimer's disease but for now let us just say that it is its own entity characterized by specific symptoms such as trouble remembering simple names of people who one may have met recently, trouble remembering conversation, and increased tendency to misplace things and similar problems whereby the individual is aware of these difficulties and begins to increase reliance on notes or calendars to help mitigate this problem. This problem is such that it continues on a daily basis in the same manner.

There is no specific medical treatment for this problem. Those affected can take memory-enhancing medication used for dementia or Alzheimer's disease, the cholinesterase inhibitors, or they can take lots of antioxidants, such as vitamin E and vitamin C, eat a diet rich in berries of all types, garlic, onions, omega-3 fatty acids, flax seed, beta-carotene, and selenium. Selenium apparently helps keep cell breakage in check, allowing cells to repair themselves giving immunity to arteriosclerosis and other threatening conditions causing dementia. Beta-carotene is another vitamin antioxidant that protects us humans from the bad effects of free radicals in our bodies, namely those entities that cause cancer. However, there have been studies that show excess beta-carotene intake can lead to prostate cancer itself. This was announced in a Swedish study some years ago. There is much that we as doctors and scientists do not know about how foods work in concert with the nullifying effects they have on disease. But we do know that antioxidants stave off many diseases that lead to early aging and chronic diseases that affect the demise of man with respect to memory and subsequent life as we know it.

Early Warning Signs

The disease of memory loss can be most devastating and differs from mild cognitive impairment associated with aging itself. Early signs and symptoms can include: memory loss that affects job or lifestyle; difficulty performing familiar tasks, such as cooking, driving, paying bills on time (of course none of us want to do this anyway); problems with language, such as forgetting common words; disorientation to time or place, including getting lost; poor or decreased judgment; constantly misplacing things; a change in personality; and loss of initiative. These are but a few of the signs and symptoms of memory loss. The disease starts with short-term memory problems, as I have stated. This escalates rather quickly and the more simple types of difficulties, like forgetting your glasses and keys, worsens into making larger and more visible errors in time, space, judgment, and orientation.

I am reminded of a situation that occurred with the grandmother of a friend of mine when she was about sixty-eight years young. The doctor told her that she had to walk a mile a day in order to keep up her health. She is now ninety-eight years young, in perfect health and none of us or her family knows where she is! She probably doesn't know either. I guess she just kept walking.

Wandering is a big sign of memory loss and is most common in dementia or Alzheimer's patients. This is one reason that most facilities for the memory impaired provide a lock-down environment for people of this ilk. For those persons bordering on gross memory losses who begin to wander, families may wish to look for a facility that accommodates this specific problem, or find a live-in caregiver, who can monitor the memory impaired individual constantly. There are some facilities that are going hi-tech by outfitting their occupants with GPS (Global Positioning Systems) devices so that they know where these people are every minute of every day. There are arguments about this procedure as many feel that this is an affront to people's personal rights of privacy, but in a memory-impaired situation this may be the only recourse short of locking people up, which I find even more inhumane. Safety is the ultimate goal here.

Chronic Disease and Aging

Aging brings on the gradual decline of the human physiology. Ponce De Leon searched for many years in vain for the Fountain of Youth, but he did discover uncharted territories and peoples. Just like this brave explorer, all of us need to continue to explore the depths of our own bodies during the aging process in order to understand the process itself, nurture the process along, laugh with the changes it brings to us, and then find ways to resist getting old—mainly, keeping your body and mind as healthy as physically possible.

A person I know aged sixty-two years, after a routine dental examination for a possible tooth abscess, recently discovered that he had a rare form of cancer called multiple myeloma. This disease is fatal and self-limiting, with death as the ultimate outcome. The gentleman in question was determined to discover what the disease was—how it caused the harm it was doing to his body—and then set out on a journey of discovery to fix the problem. He retired early from work and has been on a quest battling windmills that are real in a sense; ignoring doctors and the like who are telling him that it is futile to take herbs or try Eastern medicine or anything else for that matter, which he is actually trying. He told me that he feels better than he has ever felt in his life. Not only is he doing things to strengthen his immune system, but he is doing things to empower his mind to create an internal environment of healing.

I have never let anyone tell me how I should respond to any kind of disease or physical problem, even though they have. One experience I had was listening to my own sixth sense many years ago. I was sitting on a beach on the island of Sardinia, in the middle of the Mediterranean, where I was an exchange dentist, meditating with my legs crossed one weekend day. As the sun came up, I glanced down to notice a small brown mole or nevus on my left calf about three millimeters in diameter. This mole had a black mole on top of it about one millimeter in diameter that was a little *raggedy* looking. I made a mental note to get this thing removed when I returned home. But like most people, I got busy and forgot about the mole. As luck would have it, my wife told me one morning, several months later, as I got out of the shower that "you pinched yourself."

I said, "No I didn't, where?" She pointed to the back of my left knee, which of course I could not see. I immediately went to the large wall mirror bent down looking backward between my legs into the mirror so I could see the back of my left knee and sure enough there behind my knee, was a purple, jagged spot about three by four millimeters. I pressed on it to see if it blanched, which it did not and I said, "That's not a pinch, that's a mole and it is coming off!" To make a long story short, I went to a plastic surgeon (due to my vanity) and asked him to remove the purple spot behind my knee and another mole on my forehead, which I continuously rubbed and irritated with my glasses.

And then, out of the blue, like a lightning bolt, out of my mouth came "While I'm here, take this mole off my calf!" For some unexplainable reason my unconscious mind kicked in, and I blurted out the desire to remove the mole on my calf, which I had suspected of being a problem several months before. The doctor told me that there was nothing wrong with the mole on my calf, but I disagreed with him and demanded the mole be removed despite his opinion.

First of all, I told him it was my leg and body. Then I told him that I had sewed myself up in the Sierras once, where I was camping and tore a hole in my leg accidently catching an edge of a sharp rock. I repaired wounds on my own body enough times that, if he did not care to remove the mole, I would and he could supervise. He really liked that! So he sheepishly removed the suspected intruder.

Two days later, I received a call telling me that I had a melanoma on my left calf. I was shocked that it was not behind my knee. After the surgery, I noted that the doctor took ten times the amount away from my leg that he originally told me he was going to biopsy. He said, after the fact, that he was just being cautious; but being a long-distance runner at the time, I felt this was going to be a detriment to my running ability having lost most of my calf muscle and receiving a triple skin graft from my thigh as well. The doctor told me that I would never run again. I told him, point blank, never to tell me what I could or could not do. I ran over forty races after this surgery. I ran in pain in the beginning and I limped to the finish lines, but I finished. After several years of continued running, I blew my knee out and that was the end of my running career. I then switched to mountain biking.

Events, such as the one I experienced with my leg, or death, disease, divorce, and trauma of sorts, are all considered "significant emotional experiences." The first letters of each word spells out "see." When you have a significant emotional experience of any kind, you tend to see life differently. This experience brings your mind into the forefront and focus of change. We think and then we act differently with respect to the change.

After trauma of one sort or another, life becomes a process by which you reevaluate friends, family, values, even life itself. Listening to what someone tells you to do also gets evaluated, causing you to assess personal strengths and weaknesses, personal values, and the veracity of what someone else tries to dictate to you. No one can keep a good man or woman down, so to speak, especially one who is motivated to get the most out of life every waking moment. Never, ever let anyone tell you that you can't do something. Find out for yourself. Keep trying until you achieve your goals.

> *The marvelous richness of human experience would lose something of rewarding joy if there were no limitations to overcome. The hilltop hour would not be half so wonderful if there were no dark valleys to traverse.*
>
> *—Helen Keller, deaf blind American author*

The nature of chronic disease can lie in the fact that we just don't know what exists within us. If you consider periodontal disease for instance, one can see the nature of an unknown disease that doesn't have to hurt. This disease, which is basically pain free, is found in a high percentage of older people, who have neglected themselves by not brushing and flossing or by not going to a dental practitioner on a regular basis to have their teeth cleaned. I like to remind people that "attached to every tooth is a person," thus illustrating that teeth are living, functional organisms that serve for the betterment of our bodies.

Neglect, or supervised neglect as it were, is basically responsible for periodontal disease. More recently, it has been discovered that there is a relationship between periodontal disease and chronic diseases such as cardiac or heart disease, diabetes, rheumatoid arthritis, and some of the autoimmune diseases. Therefore, it would behoove one to keep their mouths clean and preserve the dental system intact.

In the past, it seemed to be a natural thing for people to lose their teeth as they got older; but in essence, this is not the truth, as it was not really in the past, we just did not know any better at the time. People had full mouths of teeth removed as dowries for weddings. How about that toothless bride! This was supposed to save on expenses for the groom in the future. Little did people know that this chronic condition, edentulousness, caused a decreased life span and spawned many diseases of the digestive tract as well as other diseases due to poor digestion of food and the conscious alteration of diet people were forced to eat when they had no teeth altogether. Social implications also entered the equation, as edentulous people kept mostly to themselves to keep from being embarrassed.

Some chronic diseases may be looked upon as disabilities as well, like hearing loss, blindness, arthritis, and HIV, just to name a few. Hearing loss affects over 13 percent of the population over the age of sixty-five. Impaired sight affects over 39 percent of the population over the age of sixty-five. Arthritis affects over 60 percent of the population over the age of sixty-five, and HIV is on the rise in the over sixty-five year-old group. STDs or sexually transmitted diseases account for about 35 percent since the advent of the erectile dysfunction drugs like Viagra, which have inspired many older individuals to reinvent themselves sexually. Care must be taken to protect yourself, because elders are not immune to sexually transmitted diseases. One would think that experience plays the better part of wisdom when it comes to being sexually active again in later life, as if some of us have ever stopped. Either way it is wise to err on the side of caution.

Arthritis in the form of rheumatoid arthritis is a chronic disease of aging. This disease is very debilitating and painful. The result of the effects of rheumatoid arthritis (RA) and the juvenile type of arthritis (JR) are pain, more pain, and increased pain with movement over time. Various drugs are being used to quell the effects of this disease, such as the antileukemia drug methyltrexate, which can cause hypertrophy, or overgrowth of gum tissue. Therefore it would be necessary with this drug therapy to have one's teeth cleaned at least every two months to protect against this side effect. It is also important to increase homecare with brushing and flossing a minimum of two to three times daily.

This type of arthritis, as well as osteoarthritis, can also disfigure the hands, making them ineffective for holding a regular toothbrush. A patient can then switch to either a larger-handled manual brush or a more effective electric brush with a bigger handle to help with control of the brush.

Other new drugs now on the market that are a result of genetic research are protein-like drugs that bind with tissue necrosis factor to block the inflammatory effects of RA and keep the pain down, as well as the disfigurement due to the disease itself. Enbrel is the brand name of one of these new drugs. Tissue necrosis factor is a normally occurring chemical in our bodies that is involved with normal inflammation and immune responses. The main ingredient of Enbrel binds with the tissue necrosis factor and blocks the receptor sites for the chemical so that inflammation is reduced or eliminated. This is biochemistry and very complicated genetic engineering working hand in hand.

Parkinson's disease is another chronic, debilitating disease that can eventually cause death. This disease is most frustrating because of the side effects of ever increasing tremors, the inability to think properly and the side effects of the medication that is used to treat the disease.

The L-Dopa drugs have been known to cause psychosis if taken continuously. The problem with treating this disease pharmaceutically is that the more drug one takes to stop the tremors, the more tolerant one becomes to the drug. Ever-increasing higher doses can cause the psychosis I speak of, which involves severe problems with behavior and reduced physical ability in the long run. Newer medications are on the market, but they too have their side effects. So it is a trade-off and a patient needs to find a balance in order to stabilize and treat the disease. New research on the horizon involves stem cell replacement therapy for this disease. Over time, the disease will take hold and the patient will decline significantly. This may take a long time, and care should be arranged to make sure that the patient's needs are addressed and the family is advised of the future changes. Eventual stroke and cardiac arrest may occur after long periods of drug intervention and care. This is a most insidious disease and difficult to watch as the patient goes into their decline.

> ***Helpful Hint:*** People with Parkinson's disease can practice exercises for the hands—strengthening grip exercises, writing, squeezing putty-like balls—as well as eye exercises using a Nintendo DS game unit in conjunction with the game, *Flash Focus*. Keeping stimulated is a key ingredient to staving off muscle deterioration and spasmodic hand movements.

Balancing exercises help as well. Reassurance is a good option to use in helping parkinsonian patients from becoming depressed. Also, hot paraffin wax baths for hands and feet are good to relax the associated muscles of these overworked appendages. The soothing action of prolonged heat on the muscles will relax them, help them stay calm, and recover from constant tremors. I think that frequent massage of the entire body is a necessity that helps with relaxation and muscle stimulation as well. Who wouldn't want a nice massage on a regular basis? I know I would! Have you heard about four handed massage? That is two masseuses on one: what a luxury.

Aging itself can be looked upon as a chronic condition. We age from the moment we are born. Some may argue that it is not maturity and maturation that is transpiring but for the most part it is growth and decay as a process of life itself. Chronic disease has been known to accelerate the aging process by limiting one's ability to form good immune responses to diseases of all kinds and because the nature of chronic disease is to debilitate the life-form it inhabits. Man has devised certain drugs to limit these diseases and make them take longer to affect the demise of the host organism in some parasitic fashion.

All in all, life is a system of birth and degeneration, followed by regeneration, and the same scenario. Aging is the name we give to the process, and one in which humans can relate to because of the visible changes that occur along the way and the knowledge that some day we will all die. Depending upon how we choose to look at ourselves, this vision of aging will dictate how we respond to the changes that we observe in ourselves and the chronic diseases that we may find inhabiting our bodies, now or at some later date. Two things we can do to protect ourselves during this time are to stay positive in the face of adversity and be aware of ourselves with respect to our environments.

One doesn't count illusions

nor bitter realizations,

no measure exists to count

what couldn't happen for us,

what circled like a bumblebee,

without our not noticing

what we were losing.

To lose until we lose our life

is to live our life and our death,

and nothing that passes on exists

that doesn't give constant proof

of the continuous emptiness of all,

the silence into which everything falls

and, finally, we fall.

O! what came so close

that we were never able to know.

O! what was never able to be

that maybe could have been.

So many wings flew around

the mountains of sorrow

and so many wheels beat

the highway of our destiny,

we had nothing left to lose.

And our weeping ended.

—Pablo Neruda, "Time That Wasn't Lost,"
The Yellow Heart

What I have learned from elders and peers about facing chronic disease is to challenge oneself continuously. Don't accept the fact that the disease has you, but look at it as if you have a disease and it can be managed. Positive mental attitude is important and can be reinforced by appreciating the attributes we have, the life around us, and the good that we can take and give to it. Adversity is our friend because it reminds us that there is another side to the coin, another viewpoint, and there is always a way to deal with things we don't understand or don't feel we can cope with at the time. Stepping back from the issues to analyze what we need to do is the first best step. The rest comes in its own time and space. Not to worry…savor patience …

Helpful Hints:

How to Improve Memory

PRACTICE MAKES PERMANENCE

Regular health checks—Regular examinations (medical and dental), regular medications

External reminders—Alarms, calendars, newspapers, wear a watch

Memory techniques—Mnemonics, rhymes, visualizations

and acronyms

Exercise your mind—Crossword puzzles, cards, chess, Sudoku, reading, learning or writing a poem, Nintendo games like Brain age or Big Brain

Make notes and take notice—To do lists. Keep a memory book with you

Be organized—Have everything in its place; use a diary and a regular routine

Exercise your body and eat healthy

Regular exercise should take place for thirty minutes most of the days of the week; get plenty of sleep, and an afternoon nap or rest time; decrease alcohol; cut out smoking; go dancing three times a week, for thirty minutes, minimum. If you don't dance, move in any fashion you can, for example: a stationary bike, a brisk walk, swimming, yoga, Pilates, tai chi, to name a few.

Learn to relax.

Remember, nobody is perfect! We all forget sometimes. Perhaps we are tired, stressed, or preoccupied. Worry and anxiety may themselves cause memory loss.

How Can I Help My Memory?

Some Hints for Those Who Have Relatives with Dementia

- Keep your loved one involved. Make sure they have lots of friends and give them lots of exercise.
- Keep them socially active.
- If living at home, assign them household chores. Give them specific tasks, such as gardening or dusting, but keep tasks simple.
- Give them games to play; stimulate their minds.
- Let them listen to music and dance if possible.
- Talk to others who understand the problems associated with dementia.
- Form a support group.
- Give yourself a break; look for respite care at least once or twice a week (get substitute help).
- Keep some hobbies that will renew your physical and mental strength.
- Make sure they get plenty of vitamins and minerals; especially vitamins E and C as well as the herb ginkgo biloba (for memory enhancement); use gingko in moderation; check for blood thinners, such as aspirin, other herbs with ginkgo biloba, nonsteroidal anti-inflammatories These substances need to be monitored by means of blood tests. Lots of antioxidants, such as fresh berries
- Consider behavioral therapy in the management of dementia.
- Make the home environment safe. Have a home safety evaluation by a gerontologist or a specialist in the field.
- Make sure your loved one is emotionally nourished with hugs and some form of intimacy, like hand holding or more if desired and possible.

- Deliver drugs as necessary, such as cholinesterase inhibitors like Aricept under doctors orders.
- If your loved one is a wanderer, *never leave them alone* unless they are in a locked facility or room. Trust me on this one!

Chapter 5

Early to Bed, Early to Rise

HEALTHY AGING

We wander through this life in a semi-darkness in which none of us can distinguish exactly the features of his neighbour, only from time to time, through some experience that we have of our companion, or through some remark that he passes, he stands for a moment close to us, as though illuminated by a flash of lightning. Then we see him as he really is.

—*Albert Schweitzer, German-French physician, philosopher, musician and theologian*

So far, we have covered some of the things that people maybe do not want to hear about the aging process, and now it is time to discuss some of the things that most people do want to hear about: healthy aging.

Many times, I have heard people utter the comments, "I think I've lived too long" or "I've had enough of life." I just don't understand why some people say these things, let alone feel them. I guess that is not true. Maybe these are people who are tired of the rat race and want to throw in the towel. Some people are just used to being given things all their lives and don't want to work for anything, strive for success, or even make it in the end. Or maybe these are people who have done it all and are tired of doing. I even hear people say "I can't do that," when I know they can. They just have to try. I don't know, but I do know people who have done it all, had it all, and still keep doing for others. I think that this is the secret to a long and happy life! Not just doing for oneself but doing for others.

We know the motto "do unto others as you would have them do unto you." Well, how about it? First of all, we can't be any good to others if we are not good to ourselves. So we need to take care of business, that business being you and me staying healthy and productive.

Many professionals have come on the scene in the last few years including: physicians, gerontologists, nutritionists, social workers, therapists, exercise gurus, and even chefs having jumped on the band wagon, spouting theories about healthy aging, extraordinary diets, fantastic schemes to lose weight, exercise programs, newfangled equipment to increase cardiac and body strength, and more. These individuals know that the boomers want it all now and will pay for it too.

Books galore have been written about the power of the baby boomers and how the boomer wants it all, in short order, and with a visual acknowledgment of a new person in the end. Many of these books are designed to help spiritually as well as physiologically, but what I want to impart is the concept that you must first conger up the strength from within to be strong without. Faith is all important if you believe that there must be faith in order to age in a healthy manner or to do anything really and get through life unscathed; but does that really happen to anybody? I think not.

A New Wrinkle

We can't help but go through life being touched by one thing or another in order to come to appreciate the experiences of what life has to offer and to teach us about what it takes to grow both in mind and in heart. I am thinking of a young rabbi who was asked to go to a prize fight with an older priest. When they got to the arena, the priest told the rabbi that they had tickets for front row seats. As they both sat there, taking in all that was going on about them, a young Latino fighter stepped into the ring. Going to a far corner, he knelt down, bowed his head, and made the shape of a cross on his torso several times before rising. The rabbi looked at his friend the old priest and said, "Father, what does that mean?" The old priest turned to the rabbi with a smile and a twinkle in his eyes stating emphatically, "Not a damned thing if he can't fight!"

So, what does it all mean? There are stages to development, both spiritual and in being or becoming healthy. Happiness brings on a good sense of mental health and harmony. Whether a fighter can fight or not is probably the key to his or her success in the ring, but whether someone is healthy or not depends upon many factors and needs to be examined fully.

You must have full control over the spiritual aspects of self. The ability to fight is based on will and training. Without physical and mental health, nothing is achievable. Incorporating happiness into what you do is when what you think, what you say and what you do are in harmony. "We must be the change we want to see in the world," according to Mahatma Gandhi. Starting a program of becoming healthy or enhancing your health requires discipline, commitment, a good sense of self, and the willingness to sacrifice for the sake of improving potential longevity.

Questions may arise here about those of us who may be disconnected in some way from life itself. We may find this among those citizens who suffer from memory impairment or advanced Parkinson's disease, where people's minds have disconnected from their bodies. It may be a big challenge to keep these compromised people healthy in light of not being able to motivate them anymore in the direction of self-help or sustaining their lives. To them and perhaps family members as well, it may seem futile. However, these people need extra care and stimulation to help them cope, even though they may not be aware of what is happening to them in the long run.

Many people who are not well have the desire to be well. This is half the battle, so to speak, and with a positive attitude anything can be achieved. I guess I am the consummate optimist since I have seen people, so devastated by their illness one would think they would never survive it, walk again or function again in a fairly normal manner because they had the strong positive attitude to heal.

Take a recent article I read about a veteran who lost both his legs to a bomb in Iraq that destroyed the vehicle he was in and killed his comrades. Rather than let depression set in, he chose to become both mentally healthy again and physically able. Months of rehabilitation, both mental and physical, brought him to a place where he was fitted with titanium legs and feet, which from then on have allowed him to run numerous sprints and races functioning in a fairly normal manner.

> *Ask many of us who are disabled what we would like in life and you would be surprised how few would say, "Not to be disabled." We accept our limitations.*
>
> —*Itzhak Perlman, Violinist*

The first step in getting healthy then is mental conditioning by whatever means it takes: counseling, yoga, meditation, personal coaching, prayer, or a combination of all of these methods. Secondly, the drive created by such mental acuity and spiritual enlightenment will propel most people into a state of physical health through exercise, discipline, and commitment, as I mentioned previously. So, how do I do it? Hard work! Make a plan. Set some goals. Give yourself some benchmarks: that is, some deadlines to achieve certain criteria that show you how much you have achieved in a certain amount of time. And lastly, go do what needs to be done. Part of this program includes making a strategic plan that includes maintaining a healthy diet of plenty of fresh fruits and vegetables, taking appropriate vitamins, drinking enough water, and getting enough sleep or rest.

The noted geriatrician, Dr. Walter Bortz, author of *Dare To Be 100* (Fireside Books, 1996), has recommended that those of us who wish to maintain a long life follow the simple rules of "living like a Bushman," that is, "do at least thirty minutes of sustained, rhythmic, vigorous exercise four to five times a week; eat like a bushman. Return to the habit of eating what nature first lay on our tables: fruits, veggies, whole grains and lean meats. Get as much sleep and rest as you need. Make quiet times a priority; maintain your sense of humor and deflect anger. Set goals and accept challenges that force you to be as alive and creative as possible. Don't depend on anyone else for well-being. Be necessary and responsible. Live outside yourself; don't slow down. Stick with the mainstream. Avoid the shadows. Stay together. Universal law dictates that natural order is ordained by one mechanism—a well-directed, purposeful flow of energy." Brushing and flossing daily will add 6.4 years to your life—as per Dr. Eric Shapira and Harvard University. Smile more … laugh more … hug someone each day.

Well, it's a start. Don't think that this doesn't take work or commitment: it does. Not everyone will adhere to all the dictates of this mantra. Some may go a step further and eliminate red meat from their diets. I have. Keep your dignity. This is a big one. That means try to do as much as you can on your own. Do something nice for yourself and others, daily. Keep your body clean, as well as fit, and include your oral hygiene. Make and keep regular professional medical and dental checkups. Those of you who suffer some chronic malady or disease, smoke, or take a lot of drugs due to your physical condition should see a dentist for hygiene at least every two months like clockwork. If you don't have teeth, then once a year visits to the dentist are in order for oral cancer screening and a general examination.

And, above all, love yourself. If you can do this one thing, no one can hurt you unless you let them.

Starting to learn about good mental health will also help one learn about keeping in good physical condition. You need to stay strong in order to slow down the rigors of old age. Even for those of you over the age of sixty-five who are, like the average American, watching about seven hours of TV a day, can do leg exercises from a sitting position, ride a stationary bike, lift hand weights and move your upper extremities to get the muscles stimulated and the blood flowing. And you can do all this from your favorite TV-watching chair.

Keeping a constant cardiac output by forcing blood through your heart will build stamina and help lower blood pressure as well. Moderation is the key. Being a long-standing member of the San Francisco Dolphin Running Club, I am reminded of their motto: "Start off slowly and then taper off!" Sounds good. Okay, this means work at your own pace but stay consistent. Don't be one of those people who, when they feel the urge to exercise, lies down until it passes.

Be proactive about your life, and you will find that you will live longer and be happier in the long run, although English writer Clement Freud once stated, "If you resolve to give up smoking, drinking and loving, you don't actually live longer; it just seems longer." This quote may be humorous, but in reality you may actually be in a state of chemical withdrawal from some of these habits, and time can be distorted due to the addiction itself.

Your mind is not always in sync with the rest of your physiology. Habits are formed not just by doing something over and over but by the subliminal chemical addiction to endorphins, a chemical similar to morphine, generated by the body that stimulates the pleasure center in our brains. This is what keeps us addicted to doing what we did to create the feelings in the first place. Dopamine is produced, and this makes us feel happy when it is fully expressed from our brains.

Exercise is a prime example of this phenomenon. When we work to our physical limits, the chemicals fill our bodies with a rush of energy, allowing us to do more and feel elated at the same time. Runners get high all the time from running races and doing long runs to get in shape. Research has indicated that the high one gets from exercising can be carried over into the sex drive: the more one exercises, the more one feels the urge to have sex, as well as feeling better in general. I am not saying that a seventy-five-year-old person should take up long-distance running in order to increase their sex drive; however, my grandfather was a seventy-six-year-old married to a thirty-year-old woman, and they were sexually active. He was an active man, physically fit, and apparently had a tremendous sex-drive as illustrated by having ten children, the last one sired at the age of eighty! Good luck gentlemen. Much of this will to exercise emanates from knowing that one can do incredible things, including resist disease by becoming physically fit. One will also sleep better, eat better, think better, and function better in all arenas.

Most women live longer than men. Is this genetic or is it due to the fact that women work harder, physically, than men? Or is it hormones that protect them and keep them alive longer? I think it is all of the above. Child-rearing, physical work, mental work, and an active life will promote longevity for most women. The social argument for this is that women nowadays work just as hard, if not harder, than men and are experiencing the stress that men felt as the traditional breadwinners for so very long in history. Stress is a major cause of short life if it is not coupled with activity to defuse the effects of various chemical contributors to disease, such as cortisol, epinephrine, and steroids that are all produced naturally within the body under stress and duress. No one is immune from these agents, which may very well be the culprits that cause cancer, cardiac, and other life-threatening diseases affecting us all as we age.

MEDITATION

Meditation is a way to soften the blows of stress and rejuvenate. One can do this anywhere and at any time of day. I teach and practice guided imagery, which enables people to visualize the things that bother them stresswise. People can image the stress disappearing into a large vat of their favorite color and at the same time disappearing from their train of thought and minds. Blood pressure can be brought down by this exercise, headaches will diminish, never to return, and general energy levels can be heightened without stressing the body through chemicals that may cause harm.

Meditation indicates a reflective type of thinking or thought process. *Medi* means between, and I think that a state of meditation means being between thoughts in a place that is void of everything. This is what I try to achieve during my guided imagery: getting to a place where there are no thoughts so that harmful thought processes can be moved through mental space to a place that will isolate them and eventually eliminate them from the mind; hence, creating a stress-free environment and a clear-thinking mind.

Creating a healthy space for a healthy mind requires frequent meditation in order to bring about a state of balance that permeates the entire body. When the mind is in sync with the body, we then have the ability to achieve things in proportion to our capabilities. If I am comfortable with my mental attitude and I know that I am physically strong enough, then I can exercise to my maximum output. How do people in emergency situations do unthinkable things like lift cars off of people after an accident? I sense that their minds are in perfect harmony with their bodies and they can elevate themselves, or transcend levels of strength that they may have, to levels that are unthinkable, doing the impossible, such as lifting the heavy obstacle to free someone or perhaps themselves. Our endorphins kick in, our epinephrine levels go way up, and our steroids are pumping us up for action. Yes, these are the same chemicals that can cause disease in our bodies but in times of "fight or flight" emergencies these chemicals can be helpers as well.

How does one meditate? Sit or lie in a comfortable position. Keeping feet and arms uncrossed, close your eyes and concentrate on breathing comfortably in and deeply out. With each deep breath inward say to yourself "re," and with each deep breath outward say to yourself "lax." This is the word *relax*. While concentrating on breathing, allow yourself to relax and feel your skin inside your clothing, starting at your feet and letting this sensation move to your head. Then concentrate on a color that is pleasing, soothing, and comfortable for you to look at in your mind's eye. See the color swirl and move in all directions.

Then, when you are ready and relaxed, allow yourself to see the problem that you have or the physical pain that you have been experiencing. Place this entity in the swirling colored mass in your mind's eye. Let it disappear into the color. The symptom will be gone and your energy renewed.

You can also visualize a situation that is anxiety provoking and place it in a box, closing the cover tightly. Then visualize in your mind taking the box to the sea, throwing it in, and watching it disappear from view. This will help eliminate the anxiety and restore tranquility. You can continue to relax, allowing yourself to fall asleep, or you can allow yourself to awaken from this state of semi-trance, feeling refreshed and revitalized.

Should you just wish to refresh yourself through meditation at any time, you can go through this initial exercise and awaken at will, feeling very good and revitalized. Practice this method until you are comfortable with the results. It works! Nighty night … zzzzzzzzzzzzzzzzzz.

Alternative Treatment

Meditation and guided imagery are forms of alternative medicine. So are acupuncture, massage, herbal medicine, chiropractic care, and hypnosis. More and more people are turning to these types of treatments, and more and more we are finding acceptance by traditionalists who are moving toward Eastern medicine and homeopathic alternatives.

Stanford University recently incorporated alternative medicine into their medical-school curriculum. Many Western-style medical schools are turning to homeopathic alternatives to fight disease. After all, there is over two thousand years of history connected to this type of treatment.

I personally used hypnosis in my dental practice for over thirty years. I had patients like "Maxine," who allowed herself to be hypnotized and then numbed her own hand, passing the mental anesthesia along her finger into her gum tissue so that she could have a skin graft in the mouth without local anesthesia, pain, or bleeding. She also had no postoperative side effects to treatment and healed in a shorter than normal time.

Then there was a young boy with a bleeding disorder, hemophilia, who needed a surgical procedure. He allowed himself to be hypnotized and was given a suggestion to tie a string around the blood vessels in his gum near the tooth that was to be worked on to subsequently stop any bleeding that might take place. He did this in his mind's eye, which resulted in no bleeding at all—simply amazing.

The mind is capable of doing incredible things when prompted. People who are susceptible to hypnosis are usually able to be treated with acupuncture and have it work on them directly, although acupuncture works for people who are hypnosis resistant, too. Many elderly people are taking drugs like Coumadin, a blood thinner, which makes them susceptible to bleeding when injured or operated on, and hypnosis will work great for them.

ACUPUNCTURE

Acupuncture, with its fine needles, will also work and cause little, if any, bleeding. Acupuncture works on the theory that the body is made up of energy channels, called meridians, which are similar to the nervous tissue paths in the body. There are twelve main pathways.

Acupuncture is a Chinese medical technique for unblocking chi by inserting needles at particular points on the body to balance the opposing forces of yin and yang. When yin and yang are in harmony, chi flows freely within the body, and a person is healthy. When a person is ill, injured, or in pain, the theory is that there is a blockage of chi along one of the meridians. This is a simple explanation but it does demonstrate a linear aspect to the connection of all nerves in the body.

Imagine the human ear as an inverse fetus. A variation of traditional acupuncture, this is called auriculotherapy or ear acupuncture. Points on the ear are synonymous with organs within the body. This is what I was taught in dental school to help heal pain associated with the mouth and head. If you put a needle in the ear lobe for an addiction, say, then you are working on the head region of the body. The upper, outer ear rim is akin to the spine, and so on. The ear is used for many treatments and lots of different diseases or problems. Many elderly people who are not able to be treated in a conventional way for aches and pains, take too many pills, or do not want to take medicine at all, elect to use acupuncture to treat their ills. It works! Treatments range from seeing the acupuncturist several times a week to once a month.

Taking herbal medicines in combination with acupuncture will help cure imbalances that conventional medicine is just learning about. While in China teaching gerontology, I noticed a large portion of elderly people going to traditional Chinese medical community clinics to obtain acupuncture treatments and herbal therapy. Many elderly Chinese individuals believe that this works better for them than modern medicine. Only when they find that their symptoms are not lessening will they seek out alternative care at a more modern facility. This is almost the opposite of the United States.

Chiropractic Care

Chiropractic work is another alternative medical treatment based upon the manipulation of the joints and bones of the body. I became familiar with this medical art form when I was a child suffering from asthma. My father and mother took me to a friend of theirs named Chesty, who was a chiropractor. He was not a large man per se but had huge hands and arms covered in thick black hair, which I found most foreboding at the time.

He cracked certain vertebrae in my back and neck and manipulated my spine and cranium to align my body back into a harmonious system in the most gentle of ways, earning my trust. The treatment worked and alleviated much of my struggling to breathe when asthma struck. I couldn't wait to go back again, especially when the time came that I struggled to breathe freely due to asthma. This treatment has subsequently given me much relief throughout my life for not just asthma, but for pain in my neck and shoulder, joints and muscles from overwork and overuse. Many older individuals with arthritis firmly believe in this type of noninvasive treatment to help them routinely. This treatment gives them renewed use of their hands, fingers, arms, and legs to function in a pain-free manner.

No one really knows the answers to why some things work and others do not, but if a person has the potential to believe in the treatment, this can help in allowing the treatment to be successful. There has been much research about the placebo effect of alternative medicine techniques with many individuals saying that there is no scientific proof for it at all, and therefore it does not work. But, for over two thousand years, this treatment, especially acupuncture, has been effective in treating many diseases. There is no basis in modern physiology, biochemistry, nutrition, anatomy, or any of the known mechanisms of healing in traditional Chinese medicine for acupuncture's success. Nor is it based on cell chemistry, blood circulation, nerve function, or the existence of hormones or other biochemical substances.

So why is it that over fifteen million Americans spend approximately five hundred million dollars a year on acupuncture to treat AIDS, allergies, asthma, bladder and kidney problems, bronchitis, constipation, depression, diarrhea, dizziness, colds, fatigue, gynecological disorders, headaches, high blood pressure, migraines, paralysis, PMS, sciatica, sexual dysfunction, smoking, stress, stroke, tendonitis, and vision problems to name a few?

> *The real aim of criticism is not the destruction of cherished traditions—although a due regard for the facts does often compel us to revise older opinions—but a fuller appreciation of the beauty and truth of the creative work on which it fixes its regard. The word "criticism" is derived from the Greek word "kritikos," which means "the ability to select or discriminate," hence, to decide or judge. The meaning of criticism is thus discriminating judgment.*
>
> *—Unknown*

Many naysayers of alternative medicine techniques have discriminating judgment, coming from a position of elevated ego, which creates a fear of discovering that which may be based on things not able to be defined or verified. Some people live in doubt about whatever medicine he or she believes does not work for them. In the end, these people may lean toward medicine that is science based and all it has to offer, rather than the type of medicine that is foreign to them due to their lack of understanding and ultimate acceptance of something different.

Now don't get me wrong, I am a science-oriented kind of guy and trained in the traditional American way of western medicine, but I have also trained myself to be open to alternative methods that have been proven valid and have worked both on me and for me. I have studied and used Eastern medicine techniques in my own practice. So, I continue to recommend that people keep an open mind when it comes to alternative methods of healing and maintaining total body health. There is no right answer; there is only what is right for each individual. One must learn what that method is for them and come to the conclusion that, whatever it is that they may be doing for themselves, if it is working, then it will continue to work as long as they believe in it and find it helpful.

As far as doctors go, it seems that more and more traditional doctors are dividing up the work and referring to a greater number of specialists. It might be stated that those who are learning more and more about less and less, as far as a specialty is concerned, will pretty soon know everything about nothing. One reason healthcare is becoming so expensive is the separation of generalist and specialist. Who makes house calls anymore? I know only one doctor in my community who still makes house calls, and that is about it.

Times are changing, and people can find out about medical issues on the Internet through e-health web sites, such as WebMD or Mayo Clinic.com, to name two. People are much smarter now; becoming more educated about their own health and health care; and learning about themselves in relation to disease on the Internet. Doctors need to recognize this changing fact and respect their patients' ability to make decisions for themselves about care, whether that is traditional medicine or alternative medicine.

As far as continued health goes, I am reminded of the information I found on the Internet not too long ago that compared different cultures with respect to death and dying due to heart disease. The article stated that "the Italians drink plenty of red wine and suffer fewer heart attacks than Americans. The French drink plenty of red wine and eat red meat, suffering fewer heart attacks than Americans. The Japanese eat more meat, drink much more alcohol, and suffer fewer heart attacks than Americans as well. The Dutch eat much more red meat and drink a lot of alcohol, more so than Americans, and still suffer fewer heart attacks than Americans do. The answer then, according to the article, is that speaking English is what kills you!"

> *We frequently hear of people dying from too much drinking. That this happens is a matter of record. But the blame almost always is placed on whisky. Why this should be I never could understand. You can die from drinking too much of anything—coffee, water, milk, soft drinks and all such stuff as that. And so long as the presence of death lurks with anyone who goes through the simple act of swallowing, I will make mine whiskey.*
>
> —W. C. Fields, American comedian and actor

Exercise and Diet

Since we have touched a bit on exercise and diet, I thought this would be an ideal time to discuss these topics under healthy aging.

We can't help but exercise by moving our bodies, yet what we need is enough exercise to wage a constant cardiac output for a sustained amount of time. Just like our muscles in our limbs, the heart is a muscle within our bodies that needs to be exercised. The heart beats normally about seventy times a minute. Looking at a complete twenty-four hour day, the healthy heart beats approximately 100,800 times. However, in order for it to be stimulated and conditioned along with sending enough oxygen throughout the rest of the body, you must get the heart rate up to about 120 to 130 beats per minute.

To accomplish this feat, you must stress your body by putting it through movements that cause the heart to work and the body to perspire for at least thirty minutes daily. For most people this means increasing not only the amount of exercise but the quality of exercise we do. Not too long ago, I was involved in an antiaging program with people over the age of fifty that required walking at least ten thousand steps daily at a fast pace (A one mile walk comprises about 2000 steps).

The program was called "Active for Life" and used counseling over the phone to reinforce the participant's daily exercise program.

Each person was given a pedometer, a device that clips on to the belt or clothing and measures your steps. There are several different kinds of pedometers, even those that talk to the owner to let them know the speed, the time, and distance they have walked. If you slow down, the pedometer will coach you to speed up or walk more for a longer time. I am waiting for the pedometer that sends a small electric current into your body when you slow down or if you do not walk at the pace that is recommended. This is called operant conditioning and is related to Skinner's psychological research with rats and pigeons that were trained with positive and negative reinforcement techniques to alter their behavior. The noted Russian scientist, Ivan Pavlov, also did similar research with dogs. He rang a bell and they salivated because the dogs knew that after conditioning, every time a bell went off they were going to be fed. We all must learn to listen to our internal bells, so to speak, and gauge the pace of walking with the time we choose to take our walks.

Eventually, this will become automatic and defined so that no thinking is required about the pace we have to set to get maximum output. The pedometer is a very convenient coach to have and simple to work with daily. I think that walking is so easy everyone can and should do it daily. Even people who are physically compromised can walk at their own pace, with or without the use of assistance in a cane or walker. It will give you a good chance to walk with a friend or spouse and share intimate dialogue as well, thus killing two birds with one stone.

It is important to get regular exercise, and in the process, getting to know the person you walk with daily is mentally stimulating, physically exhilarating, and helps form close social bonds with other people. This process is necessary to accommodate our need to be with others and to feel useful and needed in some manner. If you enjoy what you do, then the activity will continue.

I know several ladies who walk daily. I think their talking distracts them to the point that they don't really mind the distance, the effort, and the energy they put out in the act of walking. It is a mutual admiration society, and they have done this for years. They are some of the best conditioned people I know. They seem happier, more content with their lives, and are physically fit. Try this activity and see for yourself. Being in shape and also being happy will add to your longevity.

In conjunction with being in shape, diet also plays an important and essential role in total body health. We hear about lowering one's cholesterol and animal-fat intake. Triglycerides are most important to keep tabs on, as they have been downplayed and made to seem not as important as cholesterol in the scheme of things, but this is not so. Mono- and diglycerides form together to make triglycerides. Triglycerides, in turn, make free fatty acids, subsequently connecting to form plaque in our arteries and vessels. This specific action creates arteriosclerosis or hardening of the arteries, which results in cardiac disease. Trans fats are directly responsible for contributing another source of free fatty acids and can be found in many foods such as those delicious French fries we all seem to like so much. They can be lethal if eaten regularly.

Many years ago, when I was a chemist, I donated blood for an experiment. I was called in to see my serum, which should have been clear but wasn't. It was white as milk. Serum is the fluid that carries the blood cells, and when the blood is put in a centrifuge and spun down, the cells go to the bottom of the vial and the serum stays on the top. I found out that I did not have an enzyme that dissolved triglycerides. This forced me to read labels and alter my diet a great deal. Reading labels is a good thing to do with respect to the food we eat, since our only means of knowing what we put in our mouths is reading labels or eating only organic fresh foods. I recommend it highly. Eating foods like whole grains and fresh vegetables and lowering your intake of or entirely deleting red meat, which contains high levels of animal fats, is necessary to keep the free fatty acids to a minimum.

Regular exercise helps to burn excess calories, which come from too many carbohydrates, fats, and other high caloric foods containing sugars. Coupling diet and exercise will increase your ability to live longer and maintain a healthier life. Much of this takes conscious effort until it becomes habit, requiring the discipline I spoke of previously—changing your diet and increasing exercise. I am thinking of the old Native American saying, "Tell me, and I'll forget. Show me, and I may not remember. Involve me, and I'll understand."

So, now is the time to come to your own rescue. Go to your kitchen cabinet, take out a box of food stuff, and read the label. Go into the refrigerator and take out the containers of food and read the labels. Look at the amount of saturated or trans fat in the product. Look at the amount of sugar, which is labeled corn sweetener, corn syrup, sucrose, dextrose, or fructose. These are the things that you must learn to reduce or eliminate from your diet due to possible harm in the future. Learn what is good and what is not good to eat, especially in combination with each other. You might have a meal heavy in meat and food made with cream sauces. These form fat immediately upon digestion. Red meat also takes a long time to break down in the body, so the fats sit for a longer time, putting stress on the gall bladder and pancreas, which have the arduous task of making enzymes needed to digest these substances.

Try to eliminate foods from your diet after you look at the labels and find the amount and number of different sugars in them. Again, look for corn syrup, corn sweetener, sucrose, maltose, and dextrose—anything ending in "use"—for it is a sugar. Enriched also means made with sugars. Look for trans fats and high numbers of saturated fats and remove them from your diet. Fifty-five percent of all protein ingested is converted to carbohydrate. Couple this with starch, and a lot of vegetables, and you have the makings for high-calorie meals with a lot of fatty acids being made in the body. Just like Dick and Jane crossing the street in their stories when we were kids, "Stop, look, and listen" to what your diet is made of and what is inside everything you might ingest. Eat right, eat smart. Nutrition is a keystone of the building blocks that allow us to continue to age in a healthy manner and for a long time.

A new term in our society is *diabesity*. About 33 percent of our population suffers from Type II diabetes. Many people as they age become sedentary, spending hours on the couch or in their favorite chair reading, or watching TV or working the computer. Exercise is a word in their vocabulary, but it may not be acted upon because it requires too much effort. But what these individuals do not understand is that they need to exercise to keep their weight down, to stimulate their bodily juices, such as enzymes and organ systems that help metabolize what they eat. Many people who find imovement difficult can exercise in a sitting position, or even lying down. Overall, everyone must move. The body was not designed to be stationary and immovable. That is why we were given joints and two feet—to move and, hopefully, in a forward direction. If you need an assistive device such as a cane, walker, or wheelchair, you can still move. Maybe not as fast, but you can move.

The American College of Sports Medicine took a position in 1998 about this: "The benefits of regular exercise and physical activity contribute to a healthier independent lifestyle for seniors, greatly improving their functional capacity and quality of life." As we age and certainly for extended periods of time now, it is important to find ways to reinforce people's expectations about living a longer, more productive, and healthier life. This can be done but not alone. You need to take the reins and guide your path with respect to both eating right and knowing what exercise you can do and what your limits might be.

My ninety-three-year-old mother-in-law drinks several glasses of white wine each day; eats all kinds of meat, including the organs; swims daily; still drives a car; does her own shopping; still continues to paint as an artist, and takes care of her own home, a ten acre ranch—go figure, as this defies most all universal health laws. But she does stay active and only eats small amounts of whatever she wants. Most of us do not have this luxury, so maybe genetics has a lot to do with her longevity. Her mother was ninety-nine years young when she died. I know others of her ilk who eat no red meat, do not drink alcohol, do not smoke, do not exercise, and they are overweight to some extent but have lived into their nineties.

Statistics show that Americans spend on average almost twelve years with chronic disabilities, usually toward the end of their lives, which limit their activities of daily living. Some of these disabilities are a direct result of poor habits, poor diet and lack of proper exercise. Most of us need to start thinking of how we can change our lifestyles and still keep some of the things we have become used to with respect to diet and nurture our lives by adhering to nutritional standards that will promote better health and protect us from chronic disease, if at all possible.

> *Avoid fried meats which angry up the blood. If your stomach disputes you, lie down and pacify it with cool thoughts. Keep the juices flowing by jangling around gently as you move. Go very light on vices, such as carrying on in society.*

> *The social ramble ain't restful. Avoid running at all times. Don't look back. Something may be gaining on you.*
>
> —*Satchel Paige, American baseball player*

Throughout history many great people have died early. Many of these people did not adhere to any one theory of health or exercise. Now we have in our society the twenty-four hour gym. You can exercise at any time of day or night. Can't sleep? Then find a gym. My gym is open until eleven PM, and others close by are also open late, seven days a week. There should be no excuse for anyone not to join a gym. Walking is free and one can do this anytime, anywhere, and as long as one wants without a gym. One anonymous person said about exercise: "We work out too much. We waste time. A friend of mine runs marathons. He always talks about this 'runner's high.' But he has to go twenty-six miles for it. That's why I smoke and drink. I get the same feeling from a flight of stairs." These sentiments seem very common. Most of the population does not like to exercise. They see it as work. Their philosophy follows the idea that we work all day so we should be able to play the rest of our time.

Being older and living a more sedentary lifestyle requires that we form positive habits early in our lives. Many of us may be retired and not working anymore. These retired people are just the people that need to be active in order to live longer, more productive lives. You know it is time to resume running, jogging, or exercising when:

- You try to do a few pushups and discover that certain body parts refuse to leave the floor.
- Your children look through your wedding album and want to know who mom's first husband was.
- You get winded just saying the words "Ten kilometer run."

- You come to the conclusion that, if God really wanted you to touch your toes each morning, He would have put them somewhere around your knees.
- You analyze your body honestly and decide what you should develop first is your sense of humor.
- You step on a talking scale and it says, "Come back when you are alone."

We can joke all we want about ourselves and this is good. But we need to get serious at some point if we want to be around to see our grandchildren get married and experience other significant events that will take place in our lifetimes.

> ***Helpful Hint:*** Find a good gym with suitable hours that offers senior discounts, such as the YMCA, the local Jewish Community Center, the twenty-four hour gym, to name a few. Get a good, comfortable pair of cross-training tennis shoes that are versatile and can be used for different sports and activities. Hire a personal trainer if you can. Learn what you can do and what you should not do in the exercise room. This is important—know your limits! Wear a watch that is made to measure your heart rate (these work with a chest band that usually comes with it). Buy a pedometer. Use this during the day to measure your steps. Keep a record of how many days you exercise and what your maximum heart rate is each day. Keep a record of how many steps you take each day. Monitor your water intake and your diet. Minimize carbohydrates and sugar intake as well as alcohol. Take vitamins and supplements that help build strong bones and healthy bodies. Find time to

rest and relax during the day. Learn to love what you do and you will find love in your heart for all things, especially living.

"Life is like a snowflake, so simple, yet unique; a molecule of love expanding to infinite beauty."

—Eric Zane Shapira

What I have learned from elders who never acted their age regarding staying healthy, is just that: don't act your age. My ninety-three-year-young mother-in-law insists she is not old and does not want to be around elderly people who say they are old. My eighty-six-year-young mother is active, cognitive, drives and stays social on a daily basis.

Get in touch with your inner child and nurture that ability to run, laugh, play, walk, move, and explore, and eat things that are good for you. Enjoy life! It is okay to take a bit of dark chocolate once in awhile for a reward. Chocolate has beneficial qualities and will help give you a little more energy. It has also been touted for its ability to reduce plaque in the mouth, stimulate the heart, and act as a sexual stimulate or aphrodisiac. That is dark chocolate, not milk chocolate.

I have also learned about perseverance from my elders. Those that have the will but are not physically able to do heavy workouts still exercise. They do what they can to continue to move and sweat. Maybe this is one of the secrets of the Fountain of Youth—continuing to persevere even under adversity. I have also seen that in order to live a long, healthy life, one must be an observer; watching others who have found activities and modalities which keep them healthy. Imitation is the best form of flattery, so find out what works for others, copy them and be sure to benchmark your status and note your level of improvement once you initiate an activity you have never done before.

Keep these concepts in mind: You've failed many times, although you don't remember. You fell down the first time you tried to walk. You almost drowned the first time you tried to swim.... R. H. Macy failed 7 times before his store in New York caught on. Babe Ruth struck out 1,330 times. Don't worry about failure. My suggestion to each of you: worry about the chances you miss when you don't even try.

—*Sherman Finesilver, United States Federal Judge*

Chapter 6

Sex Is Not the Answer. Sex Is the Question. "Yes" Is the Answer

INTIMACY

When you are old and gray and full of sleep, And nodding by the fire, take down this book, And slowly read, and dream of the soft look Your eyes had once, and of their shadows deep; How many loved your moments of glad grace, And loved your beauty with love false or true, But one man loved the pilgrim soul in you, And loved the sorrows of your changing face; And bending down beside the glowing bars, Murmur, a little sadly, how Love fled And paced upon the mountains overhead And hid his face amid a crowd of stars.

—William Butler Yeats, British author, "When you are Old"

Sex at any age can be a source of intimacy among individuals; however, intimacy does not necessarily have to be part of having sex. I like to break the word down into its inherent parts: "In … To … Me … See."

Intimacy, then, is the ability of one person to let another see them as they really are. Intimacy is an expression of trust, love, faithfulness, letting one's guard down. It is sharing most secret thoughts and feelings, and above all, it is the exposure of self, the most vulnerable of things, to another.

In the beginning of any relationship, there is the initial fire that makes a sexual relationship one of passion and exuberance. As time moves forward, and two people stay together dealing with the mundane details of life and the nuances of relationships, a new look at the bond between two people brings out something what the ancient Greeks called *agape*, a deep love that leads to a sense of sharing. As agape deepens, there is a sense of sharing that develops among people who experience this intimacy in its closest form; where people can say, do or act out anything in front of another without being judged or suspect. This is love at its deepest point and finest hour.

Many of you reading this book may have experienced this love, and some of you may be just at the initial point of experiencing this phenomenon. This type of love happens after being together with someone for many years, and it can happen in the later years of life, too, after a person matures, loses a spouse, and has to start over. The initial passion might take longer to develop, but the agape and intimacy happen a lot sooner due to the maturity of the two individuals who have experienced life before in this sense.

My own parents were married for forty years. They had a love that was deep and profound. Each of them was able to be intimate with the other because of their long-standing trust in each other and each person's abilities to understand and interpret each other's signs and signals of love. I find it frightening sometimes when I know what my wife is thinking and is going to say, even before she says it. I think this kind of interpretation comes from learning about the person one is living with and the intimacy that is shared along the way. Or one might think that just living with someone for a long time gives one the ability to ascertain what the other might be thinking at certain times. It's magic!

Getting back to sex in the discussion of intimacy, we may find that sex is only a physical act and release, but it is not so much a sharing of one's most intimate thoughts. Sex can be an expression of one's love and affection toward another. If two people have an intimate relationship, then it can only enhance any sex the two may have. People should strive to maintain a constant state of intimacy, and this will help infuse an enormous amount of love, respect, honesty, energy, and willingness into the sexual part of their relationship.

Most men would like to have a partner who fills many roles, especially those that he may fantasize about. Many men tend to guard their innermost secrets and keep their thoughts hidden from a woman. This can impede the process of becoming intimate or staying intimate. A man might fear that the woman in the relationship will see him as a little boy or someone who is not masculine enough to be in control.

These types of thoughts can be profound and left over from childhood experiences. Having a bad experience with sex the first time can cause insecurity in a man all throughout his life, unless it is dealt with through counseling. Many men will not open up to a woman when they feel inadequate about themselves, and this can hurt the relationship in many ways. There may be anger and control issues in a relationship that suffers from this problem. There may be shyness with respect to sexual relations or aggressive behavior bordering on abuse that can hurt the relationship. Women can have this experience too, but it may not be as common as that which occurs in men. It can be very difficult for a man with emotional problems to have sex in the first place. The comedian, sometime philosopher, Robin Williams so aptly stated, "God gave men both a penis and a brain, but unfortunately not enough blood supply to run both at the same time."

Many men get into relationships just to have sex, while many women get into relationships for companionship. Many present-day relationships are centered on companionship, and these people may decide not to get married, only cohabitate. I see this in many older people. This kind of relationship ultimately saves money as both people share in the expenses of living together. Taxes are not increased, and pensions are not reduced when people choose to live together and not marry. There is also a mutual admiration society between both people, and every outing is a date of sorts, carrying with it new adventure and excitement. People design relationships to meet their own specific needs. Some people might opt for marriage if they are hoping to replace what they once had, but this is becoming less frequent in our culture.

My grandmother eloped when she was seventy-six years old. The family had no idea where she went, and she was gone for a week. We got a phone call telling us that she had run off to Las Vegas with a guy she met at the senior center and got married. He promised to leave her all his money if she took care of him until he died. I guess she assumed he would die first, and she married him! As it turned out, he did die first, but left all of his money and assets to a nephew none of us knew and someone he had never met himself. Needless to say, my grandmother was livid and angry with herself for never getting his promises in writing. As I have said, trust is a major factor in relationships. You need to develop this attribute over time.

Having Sex and Being Prepared

If one has not had sexual relations for some time, then it is incumbent upon him or her to learn the basics again. Many things have changed with respect to sexual etiquette, especially protecting oneself from

STDs (sexually transmitted diseases) including HIV. According to the Centers for Disease Control (http://www.cdc.gov/nchs/FASTATS/stds.htm), there is an upward increase in STDs in people over sixty-five years old. The percentage of STDs increases in the range of 15 to 30 percent, depending upon the type of prevalent disease. This is due to drugs that are used to help in erectile dysfunction (ED) among men and sometimes in women, which increase the ability of older couples to have continued sexual relations. This rather high figure also indicates that this cohort of people needs new information about the health aspects of sexual relations.

Having sex again after a long hiatus is also akin to feeling one's youth again, irrespective of the risks of doing so in today's society. Drugs like Viagra, Levitra, and Cialis help men find an erection. This does not happen all by itself, but it helps stimulate the blood supply to the penis, allowing an erection to occur in varying time lengths once the person is emotionally and physically stimulated. These drugs alone will not cause an erection. One must be emotionally stimulated and sexually aroused to achieve success with the use of the drugs. Women, on the other hand, may take small doses of testosterone, the male hormone, which can enhance their sexual desire as well as condition their bodies for sexual arousal.

These erectile dysfunction drugs have helped those persons who take a lot of different medications for conditions like high blood pressure, diabetes, depression, bipolar disease, Parkinson's disease, and dementia, to name a few. Those suffering from these ailments can now achieve erectile happiness in conjunction with being sexually stimulated by a partner. Many drugs complicate the issue of ED and the sex-enhancing value of these three drugs I mentioned helps immensely with the problem of ED itself. There are some contraindications for treatment in using these drugs, especially those people who take heart medication such as nitroglycerin and nitroglycerin-like medication. The blood pressure medications can also be a problem in conjunction with ED drugs, as the ED drugs allow blood to be shunted to the penis and this may lower blood pressure to a point where blackout occurs or even heart attacks. You should not use these drugs unless approved by your physician, and you should be familiar with the side effects of all your medications, including ED drugs.

Mind-set is important if you have not had sex for a long time. Talking about sex with your partner prior to actually doing it is important. Knowing your anxieties, quirks, likes, and dislikes, helps smooth the way to a successful experience with a new partner. If you find it difficult to talk about having sex with a new partner, then you as a couple should consider counseling in order to take advantage of a trained facilitator, who can help two individuals converse. Talking about fears or anxieties can help mitigate possible frustrations with just about any part of a relationship.

Group therapy or counseling can also be beneficial, as it provides a medium for several people to talk openly and honestly about their situations, challenges, and the like in front of others who may have similar challenges. Once people see that others have similar problems they may feel better about opening themselves up and talking about the individual set of challenges they have in light of the open communication that occurs within the group. Role-playing can help some individuals gather strength and courage to act and perform sexually when in private. Role-playing consists of acting out a series of situations that may be difficult, especially being able to talk about what one likes during sex or even getting to that point in the first place.

Several years ago, I had a client, who was ninety-three years young, with a wife, who was ninety-six years young. She wanted to have his affection, and he did not feel that he could perform adequately enough to satisfy her, so he did his best to stay away from her. Of course, he did not even take the time to ask her what would satisfy her. Perhaps just holding her and giving her a kiss would have been enough to do the trick. But he was afraid to even ask and just assumed a lot based upon his past experience, which was enough to keep him at arm's length.

His behavior frustrated his wife, and she felt rejected and unattended. So what was her response, you may ask? She escalated her requests for him to do things for her and nagged him all day long out of frustration, which angered him and lead to his not wanting to please her in any way, especially sexual. Once I found out the problem, I encouraged them to talk about their desires and what they needed to be happy with one another. After all, they had spent over seventy years with each other!

Think about how one would have to keep reinventing things to make this particular relationship interesting, exciting, and sexually attractive after all that time. But that was not what was really bothering either one of them. The main issue turned out to be just giving each other a little time and attention every day. Once those expectations were out in the open, the anger subsided, and the two lovebirds were back singing happy songs to each other again, holding hands, and kissing like newlyweds. Not every relationship ends up so definitively positive.

THE LOVE CONNECTION AND THE INTERNET

There will be a day, not far distant, when you will be able to conduct business, study, explore the world and its cultures, call up any great entertainment, make friends, attend neighborhood markets, and show pictures of distant relatives—without leaving your desk or armchair. It will be more than an object you carry or an appliance you purchase. It will be your passport into a new mediated way of life. —Bill Gates, CEO Microsoft, The Road Ahead

Many people today are meeting in chat rooms on the Internet or in dating services where they are fixed up with someone with the specifications they list on their initial request forms. There are many dating services like Chemistry.com, Match.com, E-harmony.com, J-Date.com and more, promising to introduce people to others who meet their specifications. This is all accomplished electronically.

People I know who have tried these companies have been both disappointed and happy with the results. One gentleman I know found that people were not being honest about putting up a recent photo of themselves, thereby misleading others to think they were what they looked like way-back-when. Others I know have been frustrated because after talking to their prospective dates, they finally met and were disappointed in the actual appearances of their dates. Some people explained they were a bit overweight when in actuality I would not call two hundred and fifty to three hundred pounds a "bit" overweight; I would call it excessive! So people need to really be sure who they are making dates with online.

Many times specific dating services ask so many questions of their candidates that the computer can choose a date or matches for them that are pretty much what they expected and the relationships flourish. I have found this is the case more than not, and the people are truly happy with the results. I think it is prudent to make sure you find the right dating or match company for you, which requires some due diligence and a lot of research. Remember that each one of these services is an experiment of a social nature. There are no guarantees. Also, there are Internet sites that list the rejects by people who have had bad experiences in online dating. It may be prudent to check these sites out before allowing an online date to take place.

I know older people who have insatiable desires to have sex, more than they were used to having in the past. They went to chat rooms to find mates. This activity has resulted in at least two divorces that I know of personally, where one individual in the marriage left to go off with his new Internet lover. The psychology of this action is difficult to understand. How can a person who has been married for thirty-five or forty years leave his or her family for someone they have been chatting with for a relatively short amount of time on the Internet? Most people would think that this is a very impersonal way to meet others. And it is; however, in thinking about this method of meeting, one really has nothing to lose. There is a great deal of anonymity so that people can be open and talk about their innermost thoughts, desires, and feelings in an Internet chat room. Most people find this factor attractive and nourishing, leading to a relationship consuming hours of verbal intercourse until the time comes to actually meet.

One's expectations are usually so high by this time that when the two people do meet after weeks or months of communicating and getting to know each other on the Internet, sparks fly and a physical relationship ensues. This has happened in the two cases that I know of; each new couple seemingly much happier with their lives now than before their adventures on the computer. But there are exceptions to this as well, where people leave a marriage after having an Internet relationship and find out that the other side is not all clover. Things sometimes do not work out as planned. It is about taking risks here. Of course, there are always the devastated parties left behind who must regroup, renurture, and rediscover life for themselves as new individuals.

I think part of the initial problem is that people get too complacent about life and about their relationships and take each other for granted. This, in turn, causes the relationship to eventually spoil, and one person leaves to find another more satisfying love interest or someone who can give them more empathy and understanding.

Dating after having been married for thirty or forty-plus years is very frightening for most people and anxiety provoking to the point where many people do not want to go out and explore. A person who is single, because they have lost a mate somehow, may find it very difficult to give up thoughts about the person they spent most of their time with while moving to date a new individual: they end up comparing him or her to the old relationship partner. But in order to be with someone else one must move forward and remember that there are no rules about giving up one's memories. I think it is good to compare. At least one knows what he or she wants in another. Careful planning must be set in order. *Sex 101* must be relearned with the new rules of having sex at an older age with a person you have never been with before.

> ***Helpful Hint:*** Make an appointment with your physician and have your new love interest do the same. Ask for blood tests that will show HIV status, Hepatitis B and C status, and any form of sexually transmitted disease. It is better to be safe at the outset then to be sorry afterward for not knowing these things about each other. Presumably both of you are honest enough to discuss the results. And if your intended is not willing to have these tests or discuss the results, then you are with the wrong person … sorry. There is no joking around in today's world with the increase in disease rates and even death rate among older people due to STDs. Be smart, be caring, be curious, and be persistent.

I know one woman, about sixty-five years young, who is a recent widow. She has recently moved to a new area where she purchased a new house. She started thinking about what she wanted to do, subsequently volunteering in the community. Not long ago, she had a makeover, lost a lot of weight, and started dating guys about half her age. This is what she wants to do and she is doing it. There is nothing wrong with this scenario per se, except that she is not being honest about her age. But if her suitors don't mind her age then, this is not important. When questioned, it is her opinion that "all men are only interested in a woman with large breasts and a fine derrière!" She has set out to qualify for this quest. Other qualities will have to wait, it seems. Sex is not the only object of a new relationship, but when you have gone without this part of life for so long, it is no wonder that it comes first on the new dating list for many people.

I find that people seek their own level of companionship; that is, they will find a comfortable arena to have fun in or a comfortable setting in which to go and meet others, looking for people with the same interests they have. If hanging out in a bar does not suit someone, then maybe going to a jazz club would. People must experiment to find out what is right for them. The sixty-five-year-old "makeover" visits local pubs, goes to rodeos in the area, and eats at fine restaurants in her town. Here she feels she will meet people who have the same interests she may have. On a personal note, it seems that this person is looking for physical love and not embroilment in a long-term relationship, so her choices of meeting people are limited.

My mother, on the other hand, after my father died (which would have made her about sixty at the time), went to a book club, a singles counseling group for widows and widowers, and allowed herself to be fixed up on blind dates. She eventually met men with whom she felt comfortable, but to this day she has not let the image of my father stray too far out of her mental reach for comparison. My mother's venues for meeting people were completely different than the previous example I gave about the "makeover" woman, as my mother was looking for a different kind of relationship.

Henry Ford, the great automobile magnate, commented on relationships by stating, "Coming together is a beginning; keeping together is progress; working together is success." In any kind of relationship, dating included, there needs to be a meeting of the minds, continued interest in one another, and a commitment to work together to make the relationship successful.

Honesty is an important factor here. Looking at my mother and her relationships, I noticed that she was hurt a few times in the process of dating by opening herself up to men she felt attracted to and then being let down by the fact that some of them were less than honest and open with her. It takes time to determine honesty. One never really knows another until they have spent time together. And even then, it's a crapshoot.

Love is a many splintered thing.

—Parable

Many years ago there was a country-western song with the title "I got splinters in my rear, sliding down the banister of love." This lyric illustrates the tenuous nature of love in relationships. This goes along with change and the recognition that people change in relationships too—not just a personal change, but the overall change in the relationship itself. If this change cannot be adapted to and people are not communicative about their inability to handle the change on all fronts, then the relationship is in serious trouble. It is then time for all good men and women to seek out a counselor. Learning to communicate with your inner self, understanding the dynamics, fears, dreams, and hidden anxieties about having a relationship again, all existing beneath the surface, will help clarify these entities in discussion with a future partner. This will generate a new and hopefully successful relationship for the future.

Caregivers and Intimacy

> *Do not keep the alabaster boxes of your love and tenderness sealed up until your friends are dead. Fill their lives with sweetness. Speak approving; cheering words while their ears can hear them and while their hearts can be thrilled by them.*
>
> —George Williams Childs,
> Publisher and philanthropist

I find this topic most interesting mainly because there is so little written on the subject. I have researched this for over five years and have not found anything on the topic, let alone anything worth repeating. Therefore, I have done my own research, observing couples and talking to elders who have compromised loved ones. I've inquired about how they find love and intimacy together, as well as even asking people about lovemaking when a partner is mentally or physically compromised.

I have to admit, this was a risky venture, but I was able to glean enough information so that I could formulate a list of stages to follow regarding the sharing of intimacy between partners when one or both is ill or disabled.

Over the past thirty-five years or so, I have observed many relationships that have changed due to the changing nature of the individuals within the relationship. I have seen one partner become ill with a chronic disease, while the remaining individual floundered to take care of the situation. In this situation, I have seen much nurturing going on but little intimacy in the form of self-expression and physical contact due to fear about whether the compromised person would be hurt emotionally by any advances. There was also anxiety about the caregiver even trying to get close. Basically, there was no sex or intimacy of any kind for the caregiver until after the compromised individual died or at least felt well enough to pursue the venture.

I find this very sorrowful and emotionally painful for the individual who harbors uncommunicated feelings that have been pent up, longing to come out. So what if your partner may not be aware of who you are or what kind of relationship you may have anymore? Everyone has a right to express themselves and his or her feelings for a specific person, especially one you have been married to or lived with for many years. So do it and do it now! There is no one who will stand in your way and judge you for expressing your thoughts and love to another and for another. In many cases, the caregiver, due to a lack of love and intimacy, finds another person with whom to share an intimate relationship. It is difficult to apply conventional morality when viewing this delicate situation from the outside. It is not for us to judge but to accept people's need for the basics of emotional satisfaction and nurturing.

INTIMACY

Intimacy involves some basic components such as: verbal communication; listening; eye contact; touching; hugging; caressing; whispering; massaging; breathing; lying next to one another; and the sex act itself.

When we speak of the intimacy of sex what does this mean? For starters, it means that each individual is willing and wanting to satisfy his or her partner. This also means there is a specific challenge that entails enabling the other person to be satisfied physically and, hopefully, emotionally. Sex is an expression of love and the cradling of an intimate relationship; however, for some it can be something to take up their time or an exercise for burning at least four calories of energy. Sex releases endorphins, those hormones that tweak our pleasure centers in the brain, allowing us to enjoy what we are doing and stimulating the desire to do it again and again and again!

We achieve these things by starting with the message of foreplay. A verbal message initiates the act of hugging, or just reaching out to embrace your partner is enough to initiate it if coupled with a kiss or two and some nice words. Lying next to one another quietly, simply listening to your breathing next to the other can be most satisfying. Massage is a good way to initiate sexual activity between two people as well as the stimulation of certain body parts important during the act of making love. There is also the use of hands and feet, toys, oral stimulation, experimental positions, and perhaps even bringing in a third party to partake of the festivities. All of these things must be agreed upon prior to starting, and at least one member of the couple must understand how to implement any activity between the two.

I have developed a ten stage prescription for being intimate in a relationship when one spouse or partner is medically, mentally, or emotionally compromised in some way and the other spouse is the caregiver. Talking comes first to clarify intentions and arrive at an agreement that will set boundaries that honor the limits of what each person is willing to do in the bedroom or in any intimate situation. People who care for their loved ones may wish to become intimate and have sex with their partners and this is fine. Discussing one's intentions, even if the other party does not understand, is the way to start. The soothing tone of a voice will be understood even if the words are not understood.

Ten Stages of Intimacy
- The *First Stage* is to hold hands, talk about and to each other, share your likes and dislikes, love and friendship, or your previous life together through memories.
- The *Second Stage* involves simple touching, stroking an arm or hand, caressing each other's hair and face, and talking if you choose to do so.
- The *Third Stage* includes hugging or holding, kissing each other, and continued talking.
- The *Fourth Stage* involves undressing in front of each other, with the possibility that the caregiver will have to undress his or her compromised spouse. Talking would still be in order all through this exercise. Massage could be done at this juncture.
- The *Fifth Stage* includes holding, hugging, or lying next to each other and cuddling.
- The *Sixth Stage* is the initiation of massage and checking to see if this is acceptable. This would include touching all or as many body parts as is permissible and kissing.
- The *Seventh Stage* requires everything to stop for the moment, except talking to check in, asking if everything is all right. Fantasizing by the caregiver while the caregiver holds his or her partner is an option here. Read a love poem out loud to one another in a soothing tone.
- The *Eighth Stage* begins with the initiation of some kind of foreplay, starting with kissing again and perhaps simple petting, then stopping, checking in, and continuing the activity.
- The *Ninth Stage* would be a good time to try the actual sex act itself. However, one must realize that sex and satisfaction do not require penetration, as other options can be explored. Checking in to see if all is well along the way with your partner

is appropriate, while continuing to talk and romance your partner reassuring him or her with touch and words. If there is no response, you will have to use judgment as to whether to proceed and satisfy yourself, or stop the effort. You may find that you can satisfy your partner but not yourself. This is okay and should be followed through with happiness and hugging.

- The ***Tenth Stage*** will include more hugging and holding, talking to each other with praise, stopping a moment to read a love poem, massaging each other, and kissing. Perhaps this might be a good time to initiate the sex act again. Understanding that instead of thinking of one "act," one may think of an ongoing sensual/sexual relationship that takes many forms. You should not break away or leave each other until it has been discussed and permission is given by both parties, if possible, to break apart, all the while reassuring the compromised individual that everything is all right and wonderful. Before breaking away, hugging and holding are recommended for as long as one feels comfortable doing so. Sometimes people fall asleep at this juncture, and that is perfectly fine.

All of these stages are predicated upon experimentation. That's right—it is not a foolproof method of satisfying each other unless permission is given and all the stages fall into place. That is why I refer to it as an experiment. Many people have told me that these stages work for them. I have taken the liberty to add or embellish what they have told me to the best of my ability so that the process produces maximum enjoyment, fulfillment, and intimacy.

The scenario may be different for each individual. This mechanism is just that: a way to communicate in as intimate and physical a fashion as possible when one partner is compromised and possibly somewhat nonresponsive. At least the caregiver can maintain a state of intimacy, continue sharing his or her thoughts, touching, caressing, and even having sex to a point as far as one is allowed or able to do so with the partner's permission or acknowledgment. Self-satisfaction by automanipulation is also in order for those who feel timid about approaching a partner with the thought of having sex. Whatever it takes to find pleasure and some intimacy from another without denying yourself is in order.

Many so-called "normal" individuals may have trouble having a sexual relationship with a partner who is nonresponsive. The famous British playwright, George Bernard Shaw once wrote, "I was taught when I was young that if people would only love one another, all would be well with the world. This seemed simple and very nice; but I found when I tried to put it in practice not only that other people were seldom lovable, but that I was not very lovable myself."

There may be rude awakenings for people who try this technique and get no response. They must have a strong enough ego to understand that the process I've listed is a method to enable others to be able to have intimacy with a spouse who is compromised. Also, one person may be responsible for enabling the other as well to be in touch with his or her own feelings again, feelings which may have been stuffed or lost since the inception of the change in the relationship due to illness.

> *The only thing we can never get enough of is love; and the only thing we never give enough of is love.*
>
> —Henry Miller, American author and writer

This quote is quite profound since the vehicle, love, is something that is intangible for the most part. Therefore, we express our feelings, and we should be able to accept the feelings of another. When the "other" is compromised to the point of not being able to impart his or her feelings to the one who is seeking them, that person must then be able to take solace in the fact that they, themselves, are able to make do with expressions to another, knowing in their hearts that they were received, even if nothing verbal or physical is given in return.

This attitude takes practice and great fortitude. One must learn to feel good about his or her own capabilities to tell another how they feel. I have found this always allows me to feel good when I can do this myself. One time when I did not feel good was an experience I had with my father. I told my dad, to his face, that I loved him. He did not return the comment. I was quite shocked and immediately felt hurt inside. At the time, my expectations that he would tell me that he loved me were what prompted me to tell him I loved him in the first place. It was I who was seeking the love, not really giving it. I did not realize that he could not tell me in words I so much wanted to hear, that he loved me. Down deep I knew he loved me, even though I hadn't heard the words for many years; however he was not able to say the actual words.

There was a great lesson in this, at least for me at the time: learn to love myself. Even the act of saying the words to another person means you must understand the ramifications of loving oneself first in order to be able to love another. I have since learned that I must love myself first and that my expectations should be based upon this feeling alone. If someone does not respond in kind, then I need to be strong enough to accept the fact that I told someone else how I felt, mean it, and can feel good about it.

Studying the situation allows you to understand why the person in question cannot tell you specifically that they love you or other feelings one might hope to be forthcoming. It is completely understandable to expect a person with dementia or Alzheimer's disease not to tell a significant other or someone they used to love, that they love them because they may not recognize that person as someone they once loved, or they may be at a stage in the disease process where the word "love" has no meaning for them anymore.

Some people, like my father, probably did not have a lot of people telling them that they loved them when they were children or throughout their lifetimes, and so it may be difficult for them to tell others in return. My father came from a family of many children and a father who did not speak English. My father was unable to understand anything that transpired unless it was translated by an older sibling. Once I learned this fact, I could easily understand my father's shortcomings but I did not learn these things until I was an adult.

Other gestures or phrases were substituted for showing children that they were loved, like "Do you need any money?" This is just one example, and many of you reading this book may think of other examples of how your parents or loved ones may have used word substitution for love. Even food took the place in our grandmother's and grandfather's vocabulary as a substitute for being able to say "I love you." Plying one with food always worked with my grandparents. A good meal always made us feel satiated and cared for, as well as appreciated.

All of these words and acts are akin to love in its finest hour. Of course, when dealing with a person who is medically or psychologically handicapped you may find this to be a different story. Showing appreciation or love may be the motive behind hand-holding, any kind of physical affection for that matter, babbling, constant eye contact, or even words telling one that they are loved. Spending time with a compromised individual, even without speaking, is an act of love. It is a gift.

I remember when I was spending time talking to an Alzheimer's patient on a daily basis. I would come and sit with him, talk to him, listen to him babble, and then one day he smiled at me after weeks of never having shown any emotion. I took it as a sign that he felt loved and appreciated the company and the love that I was imparting to him by spending time with him, reading to him and the like. Just showing someone that you care by being with them is enough sometimes, even if they cannot comprehend that you love someone by spending time with them. Feel good about it—you just loved someone!

> *No one cares how much you know, until they know how much you care.*
>
> —Proverb (Attributed to Don Swartz)

True Love or Scam

> *Such a morning it is when love leans through geranium windows and calls with a cockerel's tongue. When red-haired girls scamper like roses over the rain-green grass and the sun drips honey.*
>
> —Laurie Lee, English poet, "Day of These Days"

Sometimes when a person is starting over after divorce, death, a separation, or a long hiatus, love takes on a different kind of aura within the psyche. People tend to look for things they need or want and that show them they are loved or needed. Many people can become duped by love in the process and end up getting hurt. I have seen several older female clients who were taken in by men looking for sex only, when they were thinking that a long-term relationship was in store for them. The scenario goes this way: Attractive older widow meets handsome, debonair kind of guy. Usually, the woman looks for either a younger man so she can have renewed fun in her life or she looks for an active older man with financial well-being. However, there are scenarios in which men look for women in the same way.

Recently, my ninety-three-year-young mother-in-law was confronted by a man at her local swimming pool. He was a younger man and told her about himself and his passion for butterflies. He asked for her phone number, but she was put off by his forward manner and did not relinquish her number. She saw the man again a short time later in the supermarket, and he told her how beautiful she was and how enamored with her he was because her "beautiful breasts" turned him on and in the same breath he asked her for her phone number.

She was so taken aback by his comments she could not answer him. She turned and walked away. When I asked her recently if she had met any men her own age, I got this story. I decided to risk it and asked her if she felt flattered in any way by this "intruder." To my surprise she answered yes! She told me that she felt good about still being attractive to someone else at her age, but in reality she said she thought he was after her money!

This phenomenon is fashionably known and interpreted as looking for "a nurse with a purse." That is, younger men seek out older women to take care of them in more ways than one! On the other hand, several older men I know who were looking for love found women to take them in, nourish them, and eventually cohabitate with them without marriage.

I have found that older individuals would rather live with someone else out of wedlock than marry them because of the tax ramifications and benefits they might lose if they were wed. Living alone is not always a good thing if you have lived with someone all your life and now they are gone. Taking in a companion or roommate for supplemental rent will fill the void in the house; however, there are those who have had enough living with another for many years, compromising and doing for another, who now feel compelled to live alone.

Statistically, women are usually okay with being alone as compared to older single men, who have the highest suicide rate, which has been attributed to an inability to relate socially in an easy manner, especially after having been alone for some time. Women apparently have an easier time relating to others and being comfortable with the single life. Being alone accounts for a major reason many elderly individuals seek out mates. However, sometimes this can be to their detriment. On a positive note, being alone allows a person to come to an understanding with one's self. Being alone gives us the opportunity to explore life unencumbered, to experiment and try new things in life. Being alone means that we allow ourselves the privilege of making choices for ourselves and thus getting to know how we think and what we like.

Writer Eda LeShan once stated, "When we cannot bear to be alone, it means we do not properly value the only companion we will have from birth to death—ourselves."

And true to form, many people who find themselves trapped with another by choice have essentially given up their ability to make other choices, hence, failing to get to a point where they can know themselves. Being with someone because you do not want to be alone in later life should take place in a context of mutual admiration, forethought, and mental and spiritual connections. Many times, people may just settle for someone to be with because they either do not want to work at finding another soul mate, or if it comes easy, a "why not just accept it" attitude pervades.

Many people are fixed up by friends with dates with the possibility that something will click. I know many people who were scammed by the fact that one or the other of the couple put on a real good show at first; that is, romancing their partner, bringing flowers, spending money on dates, and then later on in the relationship settled into a mind-set of nonchalance, apathy, lack of attention, minimal communication, and a constant attention to the television instead of human relations. You know who you are. Now what are you going to do about it? I have advised many people to get out of this kind of relationship for the sake of sanity and freedom in the later years of their lives, when people are supposed to be enjoying their lives and not emotionally suffering because the other person in their relationship is causing them mental anguish.

The American psychiatrist, Dr. David Viscott, has commented on this kind of situation by stating, "There comes a time in some relationships when no matter how sincere the attempt to reconcile the differences or how strong the wish to recreate a part of the past once shared, the struggle becomes so painful that nothing else is felt and the world and all its beauty only add to the discomfort by providing cruel contrast." People looking for a quick love fix will find this a very common occurrence, especially if care is not taken in selecting the proper roommate.

Once trapped by a decision to take someone in but not spending enough time getting to know that person emotionally and historically can prove very disconcerting. A person may become painfully aware of the mistake made in his or her choice. Trying to get rid of the problem or mitigate the pain in some way, like asking the other person to leave, may provoke guilt, anxiety, and anger, all of which if left alone to fester will breed more anger and depression, unless of course one has the stamina and fortitude to dismiss the relationship and move forward.

On the other hand, these types of relationships can work out if people lay out the rules of engagement first; that is, communicating each other's likes, dislikes, limits, faults, and expectations. Without this kind of communication on an ongoing basis, relationships are destined to falter. Once people discuss their individual wants and needs with each other, a mutual admiration society can form with the result that each person tries to please the other and not take the relationship for granted.

Honesty is the best policy in any relationship. Getting into relationships with hidden agendas is dangerous and costly, especially at an older age when energy is at a premium and the will is limited. Why waste a lot of time suffering at the hands of someone who might have come on strong with lots of amorous talk and promises when a little prolonged communication could have exposed the truth? However, one does not know another without living with them or being with them for a while. People get into relationships on trial bases and sometimes find they are inextricably trapped and can't get out. Know before you go. This is akin to the mantra in medicine: inform before you perform. If an entrapment occurs, it is best to admit that you have made a mistake, forgive yourself, and move on without pangs of guilt, anxiety, and fear that you are a bad person. It is all about experience and this comes from trial and error.

A friend of mine recently told me a story about his father, who lives in an assisted-living facility. He was taken there after his wife passed away, and he was not really able to care for himself. He slept most of the day and pined away his time, falling into the depths of despair and mild dementia. After some time, he managed to go to the dining room for meals and started talking to people about his experiences during World War II and his later life. He was in his mid-eighties at the time. One day, after story telling, he noticed an older woman at the table who was looking at him in the most endearing way, smiling the entire time he spoke. He fancied her attention and thought that her interest deserved a return of affection. Her listening to him, he thought, seemed to pique his interest in her personally.

He developed a relationship with her after some time. I am not sure if he found out, but the woman was deaf and probably did not hear anything that he had said. But the two individuals found an attraction to and for each other because of the amount of time they spent together. Each had their own apartment in the facility, and they managed to go back and forth to see each other on a daily basis. Finally, they decided to get married. He was about eighty-four and she was about ninety-six.

The family caught wind of their plans and realized that if they married, each would lose some of their financial retirement benefits. So, they made an effort to make sure that they could be "unofficially" married and still keep their benefits. A marriage license was procured, and the part that needed to be signed by the intendeds was removed. A priest was brought up to speed on the situation, and he finally gave them his blessings, even going so far as to sign their nonlegal marriage license.

They spent several loving years together thinking they were married, until the death of the wife. This example of a relationship shows that one is never too old to find love and enjoy life with someone else. Communication is a two-way simultaneous transmission of thoughts, information, and feelings, between like forms, which when successful, leads to common meaning and understanding. Again, listening is a gift we can give to each other that is an active part of the communication process. Bingo! The goal here to be successfully understood:

> *Half the world is composed of people who have something to say and can't, and the other half who have nothing to say and keep on saying it.*
>
> —Robert Frost, *American poet*

How to Have a Good Relationship

There is no sure formula for having a good relationship. I have a few thoughts that might prove useful in the process. First, make a list about what you think you might want from an ideal mate. Try listing the characteristics of your previous partner, if you had one. Highlight the positive aspects you found in this person and place these in a new list of things you are looking for in another. Think about things you might have missed or felt lacking in your previous relationships and add those to your new list.

Draw a circle. Inside the circle place all of your values in life. Use free thinking and let your mind go. Once you have filled the circle, identify the values you wrote down with the qualities you are seeking in another. How similar are they? What differences do you observe? How will you compromise your thinking, or will you? Draw another circle. Inside of this circle write down all the qualities of your ideal relationship. Compare the qualities of your relationship ideals with the values you listed for yourself and what you are looking for in another. There should be some commonalities and similarities. Add to your master list. Be realistic. Don't make the ladder so high that no one will ever be able to climb it.

Draw another circle. Make a list of all the things you will do to make a relationship work with a new partner in this circle. This means possibly compromising some of your goals and objectives, changing your quirks and mannerisms and changing the way you do things: being open to new directions. Lastly, ask your partner to do the same exercise and then compare lists. Do not divulge what your list contains until after the other person does his or her circles and fills them in.

Once you have these things to compare to each other, you can base your relationship on some solid principles and not just on initial physical attraction and sex, although at some point these factors must be figured into the equation as well. I think that without a mental bond between two people and some commonalities in thinking, it is difficult to start a relationship anew. The information gathered within the circles gives people an opportunity to communicate on a higher level, filled with useful information that will have a direct bearing on their lives together.

> *The journey in between what you once were and who you are now becoming is where the dance of life really takes place.*
>
> —*Barbara De Angelis, PhD,*
> *American author and educator*

Again, we are dealing with change as indicated by the word "dance" in the above quote. Dance involves the constant movement of the body, predicated on a specific thought process and subsequent action or reaction. Change is constant, and when forming a new relationship with someone, we must be open to new things, changing the way we are used to doing something, learning how to please others rather than ourselves, and finding new paths to loving another—all of which are indicative of change that needs to be considered in new relationships.

Recently, I spent time listening to a woman, eighty-nine years young, and I emphasize young because she has more energy and drive than most people my age. She is a widow and takes herself on a cruise somewhere every four months or so because, as she puts it, "I like to dance." The cruise affords her the leisure time to get to know people, enjoy her time dancing on the ship, and seeing new and different venues as well. Recently, Sylvia (a fictitious name) met a debonair foreign man on board a cruise ship who reminded her of her late husband. He loved to dance, was most genteel, soft spoken, formal, handsome, and well-off. Apparently, he was everything she ever wanted in a man, other than her late husband, whom she compared everyone to constantly. There is no harm in doing so, as I have stated before, because she spent over sixty happy and glorious years with her late husband, and that is irreplaceable.

After spending time with Sylvia, the gentleman proposed to her. The answer was an emphatic "no," because she felt that he should not leave his family in another country and in no way was she moving. Because she felt so strongly about him staying with his children and grandchildren, she let her dream of marrying him go.

Was Sylvia a martyr? Possibly, but even more important to this story is her respect for family. I cannot fault her for her choice, as only she knows what is in her heart. All the criteria on her list were met, and she was most enamored with his charm and manner, but the timing was not right for her to marry him. Sometimes one has to go with "not what one feels in his or her heart but what pulls in one's head." Sylvia went on this cruise to have fun, enjoy life, to experience people and to dance; not necessarily to find a life partner.

I asked her about a relationship at her age and at this time. "How do you feel about having sex?" I asked. "Fine," she stated, "but not until I am married!" After all this time, Sylvia, almost ninety years young, still had her principles and stuck by them. We make our own rules, our own decisions regarding who we want to be with and how we want to structure the relationships we have one at a time. If you are lucky enough to have the energy and the moxy to have more than one relationship at a time, the more power to you.

When you find love, follow it to the ends of the earth.
And when you approach love, walk gently toward it, with

arms outstretched; accepting, fearless, anticipating and in nascent innocence. And when love speaks to you, listen to its calling as the warmth from its being envelopes your soul as a great fog. And yet, be cautious when the knowledge of love's breadth brings you closer to its grasp; in that love can be a blessing, bringing happiness or an embedded thorn, causing pain.

—Eric Zane Shapira, "On Love"

And then, there are those who joke about individuals who have been married numerous times. Questions arise like "Why can't you get it right?" and stories, like the one about a woman who was married seven times: her first six husbands died of mushroom poisoning, while the seventh and last husband died of a brain concussion, all because he wouldn't eat the poison mushrooms!

When it comes to marriage or relationships in general, choice is the operative word and taking responsibility for your choices is the bottom line. Setting up a relationship of any kind requires taking responsibility for the choice and making sure that your commitment to the relationship is understood. We do this through good communication, not making false promises. We do this through our actions, backed up with solid facts, often verified in writing, such as an agreement about our type of relationship: who will own what property and what will happen if one party chooses to move on and leave the relationship? There is nothing wrong with getting things in writing to protect yourself at the outset. Prenuptial documents are good to have when considering marriage, and protecting personal property is a must, especially personal property that has been handed down for many generations.

I know a man who, when first married, had an agreement with his wife that if anything ever happened to their relationship, her wedding ring was to be returned to him. The diamond belonged to his great-great-grandmother, and his grandmother gave him the diamond with the stipulation that it remained in the immediate family. When the marriage ended in short course, he realized that he had only received a verbal agreement about returning the heirloom ring and nothing in writing. All hell broke loose in his mind thinking that he would never get the ring back! He finally did retrieve the ring, but it cost him dearly in money he did not have at the time. So, it is a must to consider, irrespective of personal pride and all else, setting up a written agreement in a legal way to keep property apart if something should happen to one or the other of the parties concerned. It was a hard lesson for my friend to swallow; one I wouldn't want to see anyone else have to experience needlessly.

What have I learned from older people who never acted their age with respect to love is that love or the quest for love never dies. As if one were Don Quixote looking for love, so shall all of us live our lives. The entity of love is one that sustains us, keeps us sane, for the most part, and gives us the nurturing that we as humans so need and desire. Just because someone is over sixty-five does not mean that love is not in the equation of life anymore. Just because someone has lost a spouse of many years or is divorced does not mean that they do not deserve to love again or cannot seek love elsewhere.

First, you must love yourself, and secondly, you must learn to share that love with others who can share their love in return. It is give and take in all respects. Above all, love should not be blind. Follow your feelings, yes, but don't allow them to blind your sense of responsibility, good judgment, and sense of self. Rule number one is to love yourself. This fact is a priori to everything else. You must learn to do this if you feel that you cannot love yourself or don't know how. Self-love is an appreciation for who you are as a person. Self-love is an expression of inner gratitude about what you have accomplished in your lifetime and what you have shared with other people.

I have learned from older people to love myself, and I have come to appreciate myself as an integral part in this world. I am not trying to compete with anyone. I only compete with myself and try to become a better person as I go along. There is always room for improvement. Fine wine improves as it ages, why not individuals? I see the beauty in older people as they seem so sure of themselves for the most part. Sure, there are those who are lost or compromised in some way, but there is still beauty in them and what they have accomplished and continue to accomplish. We can all be one of these people if we keep our faith and interest in ourselves and our self-love real and up to date.

The heart that loves is always young.

—*Greek Proverb*

Chapter 7

To Be or Not To Be—Families in Crisis

Anxiety is essential to the human condition. The confrontation with anxiety can relieve us from boredom, sharpen the sensitivity and assure the presence of tension that is necessary to preserve human existence.

—Rollo May, American psychologist

Families in crisis can mean a lot of things in our modern society. All crises create anxiety for the people involved. Anxiety is predicated upon some kind of previous experience that has had a profound effect on us, so much so that mental "tapes" have formed in our brains. The memory bank of trauma, no matter how big or how small, when activated, brings about chemical and physical symptoms we label as anxiety provoking.

So what is crisis all about? It can be nothing more than where did I leave my wallet? That kind of crisis sets up an immediate fight or flight syndrome in the body, causing specific organs to secrete their internal potions, which in turn may cause the body to feel nervous, excited, and sweaty with heart palpations and dizziness. These physical symptoms, combined with the loss of mental acuity, lead to the state of anxiety.

A New Wrinkle

Anxiety, then, heightens our state of awareness, allowing us to react to the stimulus that provoked the situation in the first place. This mental state leads to the message "let's go find the wallet." No matter what the situation, the chemistry is pretty much the same. The reactions may be different depending upon the previous experience, training, and one's ability to handle crisis when it happens. Good judgment is important here, and this also comes from previous experiences that involved poor judgment. It is a circle of sorts.

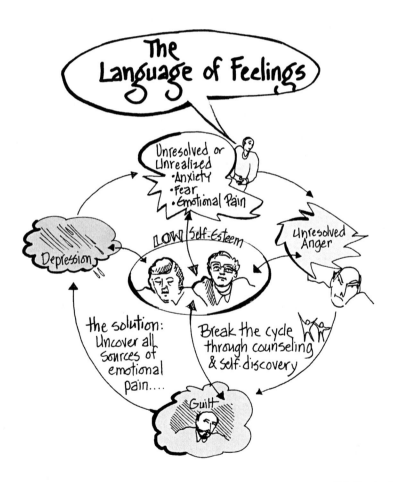

© E. Shapira 2009

When families experience crisis connected with an aging issue, this anxiety may not be credited to any prior experiences but may be a void where no previous experience exists. Therefore, having no information or knowledge about how to handle an aging issue or crisis will inevitably create anxiety, leading to a family in crisis. At this juncture, it will be important to know where to go to get the information that will assuage anxiety and help make the experience a much more tempered one, however, not without paying respect to the symptoms one feels because of the anxiety itself.

A gerontologist is more than likely a good choice when it comes to handling the challenges that the aging process brings about in a sometimes sudden manner. Recently, I had a call from a woman who has a ninety-five-year-old mother. She complained about how anxious she has become because her mother is senile and suffers from dementia. Within this disease lies the possibility of uncontrolled libido and acting out of emotions. The mother is now telling her daughter how much she hates women and how she does not want to be around them, including her daughter. This makes the daughter ineffectual as a caregiver and has generated anxiety and the need to find someone to help her. There are drugs that can help with this problem, and some of the hallucinations the mother has as well, but it will be up to the daughter and her husband to decide if this is the way they want to go, or if they might hire a male caregiver to help the mother. Either way, they will suffer from anxiety until the problem is resolved in a manner that they are mutually satisfied with.

Family crisis can be a good thing because it will stir the family to act rather than have them sit complacently by, waiting for the problem to rectify itself or the person who has created the problem in the first place to go away somehow—perhaps dying. I know this might be a callous thing to say, but it is all too often the truth. Rather than let themselves be stressed by an aging relative and his or her problems, people sometimes just wait it out until death occurs.

Most people find it prudent to seek help in one form or another. They may wait for the person's physician to get involved and help them or they might ask friends if they have had a similar experience. In this case, asking friends, one gets answers to a situation that might seem the same but in actuality was different, in which case there is no panacea. What happens to the next guy might happen to you but in a different way and with a different solution.

Crisis may be defined as "a time of great danger or difficulty." It is also defined as "a turning point." Indeed, the Chinese word for crisis also means opportunity. So, by looking at the problem as an unmet need, one can find an opportunity for positive change.

Not too long ago I had a client who was struck down with cancer. Her daughter came to me in a frenzy, full of anxiety and stress because she found herself with the responsibility of taking care of her mother, while at the same time having to give up some of the things she liked to do in her spare time, like exercise and dancing. I knew there was a way around this and suggested a caregiver who could take care of Mom during the day, when the daughter worked, and then periodically at different times during the week in the evening so the daughter could do her thing. This worked out well, great for the mother and the daughter, even giving the daughter some free time to sit with her mother, sharing quality time with her, all along knowing that the caregiver was there to help with the house, the meals, and whatever else was needed. During this stressful period, the daughter learned to relax and trust me and others with her mother. Having quality time with a loved one is a gift, especially when one is facing cancer and the possibility of imminent death. Being moved into action by necessity is what crisis does for people. I think that with every crisis comes a learning period. We tend to learn what we need to do in order to get over the crisis, which results in learning much more about ourselves with respect to our limits and our abilities to handle stress. Crisis involves change and action.

Charles Edison, the son of inventor, Thomas Edison, in a December, 1961 Reader's Digest issue wrote an article, "My Most Unforgettable Character," discussing the stress and crisis of his great inventor father. One can see that through severe adversity and crisis, people can rise to the occasion and perform acts that bring positive change to themselves and to humanity. According to Charles, "Thomas Edison devoted ten years and all of his money to developing the nickel alkaline storage battery at a time when he was almost penniless. Through that period of time, his record and film production company was supporting the storage battery effort. Then one evening the cry of "Fire!" echoed through the plant. Spontaneous combustion had occurred in the film room. Within moments all of the packaging compounds, celluloid for records, film, and other flammable goods had gone up with a whoosh. Fire companies from eight towns arrived, but the heat was so intense and the water pressure so low that the fire hoses had no effect. When I couldn't find Father, I became concerned. Was he safe? With all his assets going up in smoke, would his will be broken? He was 67, no age to begin anew. Then I saw him in the plant yard, running toward me.

'Where's Mom?' he shouted. 'Go get her. Tell her to get her friends! They'll never see another fire like this again!' At five thirty the next morning, with the fire barely under control, he called his employees together and announced, "'we're rebuilding.'" One man was told to lease all the machine shops in the area, another to obtain a wrecking crane from the Erie Railroad Company. Then, almost as an afterthought, Edison added, "'Oh, by the way. Anybody know where we can get some money?'"

Virtually everything we now recognize as a Thomas Edison contribution to our lives came after that great disaster. And so be it, from crisis to persistent solution in one breath. Just think about how many times Edison reworked the invention of the light bulb—approximately 114 times! This alone would create enough anxiety in most people to cause a nervous breakdown. But Edison's attitude was that "there was no failure, only results." He stated, "I haven't failed, I've discovered one more way on how not to make a light bulb."

There are many examples like this one, but none as surprising as Edison's ability to regroup and move on through adversity as if it never happened. People need to be flexible through crisis and open to new ideas if they are to mitigate the stress and anxiety, and change the situation to a positive one. Age is both irrelevant and necessary for the experience to make a difference.

FAMILIES IN TRANSITION

Families who are brought together by crisis find themselves in transition. The transition of aging and the transition as a family being forced to communicate in serious terms as well as in a logical and orderly manner are difficult positions to be in, while the person who caused the family to come together in concert is waiting for care. In order for anyone to wade through the anguish of crisis, they must first define what makes up the crisis at hand and then set goals to get around or over the crisis in a manner that will be successful for all concerned and one that will be rewarding in a personal sense for all participants. We can't have the person who is waiting to be rescued from despair sitting around wondering if anyone will answer the prayers and concerns he or she has or letting them think that they are alone for any great length of time. This is not acceptable.

So the first response to crisis is to verify the cause and effect of the emergency and then categorize it in terms of how it will be delegated in order to handle it effectively. Next, brainstorm ideas to solve the situation, all the while letting the person in crisis know that their concerns have been heard and are being worked on. You must also set a time line for getting back to the person in crisis with suggestions on how to solve their problem or unmet need. Sometimes it is very difficult to rationalize a good response to a crisis with an older individual who suffers from dementia, because they may be too emotional or incoherent to understand.

In order to set a goal around a crisis several steps must be taken to ensure proper thought and eventual action toward that goal.

Be **SMART** when goal setting, meaning, make your goals:

S—Specific

M—Measurable

A—Attainable

R—Relevant

T—Time-bound

I think that being specific about a crisis means being able to define the problem or unmet need in an understandable manner. You must be able to understand the challenge as it relates to the person who is exhibiting the problem and try not to understand the situation only from your own perspective. This way, by putting yourself in another person's shoes, you can walk a mile first in order to ruminate on the ways this person is experiencing emotional or physical discomfort. You can then come to some conclusions about setting your plan in action to relieve them of the burden.

Finally, when you do come to a conclusion and hear that the projected plan may not be satisfactory or warranted in the eyes of the beholder, you are at least a mile away from the mayhem you have possibly created by trying to make a plan that was not good enough in the eyes of the sufferer. And then you can take satisfaction that you have left the other person barefoot and not able to catch up to you for retribution!

Now, consider the advantage of technology, which is a good thing, especially having a cell phone. You can call in your solutions.

Next, in order to make sure that the goal is attainable, your objectives to fix the problem should be measurable and charted. These objectives can be timed so that the benchmarks will provide an adequate path to follow. Attainable goals are good and make it easy for all concerned to achieve success. This will help eliminate the possibility of frustration and help create unity of purpose among all those who are involved in trying to help solve the problems.

Having a relevant goal is important so that there is no wasted time or energy involved with the situation or problem. Too many times we are bombarded with ideas from family members about how to solve a problem in a certain family situation that suggests a self-directed and self-motivated objective. This selfish act can hurt feelings and inject anger into the communication process, which leads to guilt, anxiety, and failure of purpose. This type of thinking definitely disrupts family dynamics.

Lastly, having a unity of purpose will allow you to stay time-bound and on track to the finish line. The problem will dissolve, and in analyzing the situation you can see that by having an organized process the crisis can quickly be rectified.

Sometimes the problem is not rectified because there are too many differences of opinion, and this is when a clinical gerontologist or counselor of some type should be enlisted to help. This gerontologist has developed a system by which families can come together in peace and learn to take responsibility for their part of the family's unmet needs. It is always difficult to accept that there is a problem occurring when one is not close to the situation. In this scenario, judgment is passed that may skew the other family members' perceptions about the black sheep in the family and communication may subsequently fall short between the siblings and parents or parent involved. Bringing families together is what good processing is all about.

Not too long ago I was asked by several siblings to come and see their mother due to increasing subtle changes in her thinking, memory and attitude. I asked that the siblings be present as well when I interviewed their mother for the first time. I did this because I wanted to get the entire picture of what I was going to be dealing with and who was involved here. Each sibling had a different role in their mother's life. Each daughter had a specific job but was not giving the mother all the information she needed at the time and this created stress for the mother. The stress manifested itself in memory loss, anger and feelings of resentment. I subsequently asked each sibling to look at their mother as the head of the family corporation, which in reality she was. But my motives were for support. Each daughter was asked to support the family corporation by allowing the mother to have her own opinions and also to inform the mother about what was going on in the corporation, from their standpoint, on a daily basis.

I set up a mock corporation, making each sibling a stakeholder in the corporation and giving each one a chance to set their priorities around their mother, the actual business of the corporation. This worked very well, as each sibling took a role, made agreements with the others, and communicated their desires for each other and for Mom. I had them each write their job descriptions and the commitments they each were willing to make on paper. It was a very successful outcome. Having each person make a commitment to take responsibility for his or her mother was the trick here, especially doing so in front of each other and God.

> *If you want children to keep their feet on the ground, put some responsibility on their shoulders.*
>
> —*Abigail Van Buren, Columnist*

You may find it extra difficult to convince the black sheep of the family to powwow with the rest of the family, since he or she may have their own ideas about things or not care at all about anything but him or herself. Asking for help from the reticent one will usually do the job. This act shows trust in this person's opinion and their importance within the family. It must be stressed that this person's input will be regarded in the highest of esteem during the discussions about the problem at hand. However, as the late comedian and actor, W. C. Fields once stated, "If at first you don't succeed, try, try again. Then quit. No use being a damn fool about it." Sometimes it is not worth the final effort to get a slacker to yield to family desire. It is at this point that one must cease all efforts that might injure the totality of the remaining family dynamic.

FAMILY DYNAMICS

How does one develop a good family dynamic you might ask? The family must enter into negotiations in order to define what the objectives of the unit are toward being successful in its endeavors. That is, set a mission statement for the family and look toward a vision statement, as well, based on the core values of the family. I know this sounds involved and serious, but it is a necessary step in order to achieve unity among all the family members. Deciding what the family is about is important when it concerns a family member and the overall family in crisis.

Auditing the family members for specific skill sets will help determine responsibilities and create an action plan. Each family member must set personal goals around the person in the family who needs the help. That means defining how each person will commit to helping the individual and, in essence, helping the family. The family must decide who will be the spokesperson for the family and the backup spokesperson if handling challenges alone becomes a burden. Going around the table to determine each person's perceptions about the others can be most illuminating for the family. After learning who is doing what and when, the family can begin to set goals for the person in need and move forward with an action plan.

Each person needs to understand themselves and their own abilities with respect to doing something for the family member in crisis. This takes serious reflection and thought. Meditation may be in order or even counseling so that thoughts may be exposed that even the person being counseled had not considered before. Questions concerning self skills, recognizing skills in other people, developing trust in others, discovering what will be a satisfying result, and exposing all hidden agendas and expectations will come out of much pensive work either alone with guided direction or with counseling and direction. The family dynamic will be strengthened once these discoveries are made about each person in the family. Happiness will be restored as well.

In another example, a gentleman became somewhat lost due to cognitive impairment—lost in the sense that he started making decisions on the spur of the moment and lost his libido to the point of being belligerent, angry and abusive to his wife and daughter. His wife placed him in a facility because she could not take the abuse anymore. She then became depressed, in turn causing a chain reaction among her daughter and the daughter's family as well. It was like lining up dominos, flicking one and watching the rest fall, one after the other. The daughter saw my name in a local magazine ad and called me to help out. I had the daughter and mother sit with me and answer some questions as well as a filling out forms that asked about their fears and values. Each one had a different set of concerns and each one on hearing the other's comments broke down in tears. The question at hand was, "do we leave Dad in a facility and what kind?" Once the family was clear on each other's feelings and came to some kind of agreement on what had to be done to help Dad, and Mom as well, they could move forward with making a plan. This helps take people out of the stress they are in due to not knowing what to do. Some of you reading this material may find yourselves in a situation that is similar in substance and at a loss as to where to start, just like these people.

If you don't know where you are going, any road will take you there. Follow my method for setting goals by brainstorming ideas and making an action plan. Call a gerontologist to help. Write your thoughts down and think in a logical manner, and you will be able to come to a consensus about what to do and how to do it. Otherwise, you will have to find another way to deal with your can of worms. Zymurgy is the last word in the English language dictionary. Its meaning is synonymous with the study of fermentation. The society of fermentologists has coined several laws to describe the process. Getting into trouble or getting lost in a process sometimes creates a can of worms for most of us. The Zymurgy Society's First law is as follows:

> *Zymurgy's First Law of Evolving System Dynamics: Once you open a can of worms, the only way to re-can them is to use a larger can.*
>
> —*Zymurgy Society, Conrad Schnieker, Member*

SWOT Analysis

It is most important that families understand that there is a need to be organized in planning for crisis. One does not want the shoot-from-the-hip kind of response when dealing with a situation that encompasses more than one person in the decision-making process. Therefore, it is incumbent upon the family to learn how to implement direction for change by using a SWOT analysis in their planning. The SWOT analysis deals with the following entities:

Strengths

Weaknesses

Opportunities

Threats

These words each stand for an avenue of awareness that you will need to embark upon with respect to your own abilities and the abilities of the family to problem solve. Once these headings are understood fully by defining what it is that makes up these categories, families can then move on to an action plan by setting goals.

> *It is probably not love that makes the world go around, but rather those mutually supportive alliances through which partners recognize their dependence on each other for the achievement of shared and private goals.*
>
> *—Fred Allen, American comedian*

Once the SWOT material is in order, you can use the information to set both long-term and short-term goals, followed by determining objectives that support the goals. You should prioritize the objectives and define and detail them by placing them in a diagram of sorts—a flow chart—which will illustrate a pathway and direction to follow. Then, you can put the plan into action by implementing your objectives in an orderly fashion and, afterward, analyzing your results and determining the outcome in the form of an evaluation for each person in the family, their performance, and the progress of the individual's and family unit toward the major goal of eliminating or alleviating the crisis at hand. SWOT only works if people in the family are honest with themselves and each other. This will promote trust and determine each person's comfort level with the others, both in and out of the group.

Healthy family dynamics are necessary in order to achieve any goal, because without family cooperation, feelings of mistrust, anger, jealousy, and bad rapport may result. This potpourri of negative feelings will disrupt the business at hand and delay any type of positive problem solving. Work of this nature only gets more difficult as we age, and we find ourselves leaning in the direction of becoming set in our ways. Therefore, it is best to learn and utilize active planning techniques early in life so that these techniques become second nature to us as we reach older age. It is imperative to remember to allow yourself the flexibility to be open to change. An old proverb states that "when you change your direction, you change your world." It is also important to remember that when working with other people that they may have different agendas then you do. In this case, you need to respect everyone's point of view in a nonjudgmental way, remembering that a positive result is what you are all working toward.

> *Kind prince, to have integral virtue is to have unchangeable virtue. In daily life, one should fulfill one's obligations in the five great relationships. As a parent, one should love one's children. As a son or daughter, one should abide by one's*

> *parents' deep wish for one to live a decent, healthy life. As a subordinate, one should carry out one's duty unfailingly with a sense of cooperation and teamwork. As a superior, one should assume full responsibility without blaming one's subordinates as an excuse. As a brother or sister, one should extend love and help to the younger ones, and the younger ones should to the same for the older ones. AS a friend, one should be faithful. AS a husband or wife, one should devotedly care for one's mate. In general, one should carry out any work that comes to one with righteousness. One should be concerned with making one's best contribution rather than seeking unrightful promotion and personal profit. One should practice steadfast and indiscriminate virtue without demanding others to do the same in return. These mental attitudes are the manifestations of such virtue.*
>
> —*Lao Tzu*

Transitioning the Transition

I remember my father's words around the house when I was a child; inevitably he would respond harshly to my doing something he felt was wrong. I can still hear him telling me "There is the right way, the wrong way, and MY way!"

It seems all too often that getting over the hump is a difficult thing to do. Don't give up! Working with others can be fun and, yes, challenging at times, but the rewards are great. Overall, you must think about the person in crisis. We must come to a consensus prior to acting on the plan. Mobilizing is difficult and can take a lot of time and energy, which in essence takes time away from the person in need.

The importance of short-term goals here cannot be overemphasized. One needs to have a short-term plan of action based on these goals in order to act on the long-term goals and plan. Therefore, it is necessary to work on both fronts at the same time, planning what needs to be done with the information as it is gathered. Using family for these tasks is important. That is why it is important to know what each person is capable of doing and then encouraging them to do it.

> *Plans are worthless, but, planning is everything. There is a very great distinction because when you are planning for an emergency you must start with this one thing: the very definition of 'emergency' is that it is unexpected, therefore it is not going to happen the way you are planning.*
>
> —*General Dwight David Eisenhower*

Building a structure takes much planning: conceiving the project, choosing of the people to do it, filing the permits, choosing the materials, and then building the edifice to completion. Once the family decides on a course of action it can be a reality. Building something without planning is a formula for failure. You might as well wear a blindfold and walk through a yard filled with poisonous snakes! It is imperative to understand the stressors before acting on them. Take the time to isolate what these stressors are and break them down into smaller, workable parts, whereby one can complete the journey by using the pieces as stepping stones to the completion of the whole.

I had a call from a woman whose brothers and sisters decided that it was time for Mom and Dad to move into an assisted-living facility. This was the first my client had heard of the siblings' wishes and she was most distressed. Processing her expectations meant she was adamant that her parents should stay independent and remain in their home. This thinking was a projection of her own thoughts about what she would want for herself. My client even told me that the older sister, who had the power of attorney, was going to allow a younger sister to move into the parents' home after they were moved out.

My client was angry, sad, and ready to fight. I reassured her that there was a way around this and she needed to do some planning with me so that she could take the necessary information into the meeting with her brothers and sisters. We planned for several different scenarios, and she took them to the family meeting. By the way, the older sister opted out of having me facilitate the meeting because she felt I was too threatening since they did not know me. I was okay with this because my client and I had planned many scenarios, all of which would have had a favorable outcome as long as the family agreed.

The family met and my client presented her plans to the family. They hashed over all of the options, choosing one that was agreeable to everyone. The parents stayed in the home until one of the siblings found a satisfactory facility for the parents to live in. My client's brother was a businessman and a fair judge of facilities. The older sister, who was an attorney, filed all the legal documents to get the house on the market as well as other property. A trust was set up for the funds to be placed into that would cover the expenses of the parents while they were still alive. The property sold in less than a week.

My client was a happy camper because she was allowed to plan ahead of time assuring her that no matter what option was chosen, the outcome would be acceptable as long as everyone agreed—which happened. A happy ending was achieved for all.

This type of result can be yours if you adhere to a proper plan. Remember the five P's of planning: Poor Prior Planning Promotes Phailure. Okay, I can't spell, but I know what I am talking about here.

I have been there, done that and got several T-shirts in the process. Trust me on this one.

> *Let our advance worrying become advance thinking and planning.*
>
> —Sir Winston Churchill, statesman

What I have learned from older people who never acted their age about families in crisis is that no matter what age one may be, crisis can strike when you least expect it to do so. One must be able to think rationally and not allow oneself to be overly emotional to the point of being paralyzed in making decisions about a specific challenge or set of stressors.

Understanding what it is that is creating a specific unmet need is first on the list. Then, dissect the problem to understand what caused it in the first place and make a plan to correct the situation, in increments if necessary. The wisdom of older people should be embraced, respected, and utilized to help solve not only their own problems but the problems of other family members. It is important to remember to include the thoughts of those who bring their challenges to the table if they are able to communicate them in an understandable fashion. Leaving out the people with the initial problem is a no-no and will cause a backfire in the process if you try to solve a problem around an individual without including them in the decision making. Include everyone and respect everyone's thoughts. Then do what is right for the situation. It is a process that continues as long as you are a responsible family member.

> *Informed decision-making comes from a long tradition of guessing and then blaming others for inadequate results.*
>
> —Scott Adams, American cartoonist

Chapter 8

Now I Lay Me Down to Sleep

DEATH AND DYING

Memorial Day was over now; all had left and I was alone,

I began to read the names and dates chiseled there on every stone.

The names, which showed whether it was Mom or Dad or daughter or baby son,

The dates were different, but the amount was the same; there were two for everyone.

It was then I noticed something; it was a simple line.

It was the dash between the dates placed there; it stood for time.

The dates there belong to God, but that line is yours and mine.

It's God who gives this precious life, and God who takes away.

> *But that line between He gives to us to do with what we may.*
>
> *We know that God's written the first date down for each and every one.*
>
> *And we know those hands will write again, for the last date has to come.*
>
> *We know He'll write the last date down, and soon, we know, for some.*
>
> *But upon the line between those dates, I hope He'll write, "Well done."*
>
> —*Lucille Britt, "The Dash Between the Dates"*

There has been much said and written about death and dying, but most of us live in denial around the subject, until it gets close, that is. Fear of the unknown, the lack of perception about what death is and how it happens, what it feels like as well as when it will happen and afterward are all part of expecting the worst at a time when one can least afford to have it happen.

Woody Allen has been quoted as saying, "It's not that I'm afraid to die, I just don't want to be there when it happens." We all think that death and dying are painful, so we block them out of our minds. This allows us to really be somewhere else in the face of death and the fear it creates. Most of us never think that it will happen to us, at least at a young age, so why think about death at all? When it hits home by having a parent, sibling, or relative die, then the thought of not being immortal materializes and awakens us from our deep sleep of denial.

A noted researcher in human cognition, Dr. Heinz Von Foerster, once stated to me that, "If dying was that bad, people would have come back from the dead. As it stands, no one has returned as far as we know.

And no one really knows what it is to die, no one has come back to tell us how great or how bad it really was for them." As far as anyone knows, dying is a process, and death, like dying, is an individual event. Each of us experiences this phenomenon in our own way, in our own time, and at whatever age it happens to us.

> *Strange—is it not?—that of the myriads who before us passed the door of Darkness through, not one returns to tell us of the road which to discover we must travel too.*
>
> —Omar Khayyam, *The Rubaiyat*

Some of us live a long, healthy, productive life before we die and can claim many accolades. Others die at a young age, having hardly experienced life as most of us will know it or experience it. The *Oxford American Desk Dictionary and Thesaurus*, Second Edition defines death as an "irreversible ending of life; an event that terminates life; being dead; a destruction or permanent cessation." This definition is quite definitive as far as one who will not live anymore. Does this mean that a person who does nothing is dead? I guess that is semantics. And one who is going through the dying process then is essentially dead, because that person is experiencing the termination of his or her life as they know it.

In light of a philosophical discussion about what is death and when is one actually dead, we will say for all practical purposes that when one ceases to live by breathing, functioning in a normal physiologic manner, or essentially being brain-dead, they are dead.

Psychiatrist and author Elizabeth Kubler-Ross developed the theory that includes the stages of dying, but in her later years as she was dying herself, she as well as others repudiated these stages as a fabrication. According to various other psychiatrists in her time who had different viewpoints, her observations were found to be "simplistic, monolithic and not germane to all." The stages included: denial, anger, bargaining, depression, and acceptance. Not everyone abides by her theory or follows the stages of dying that she set forth in her theory.

My own father became very angry when he discovered at the young age of sixty-one that he had lung cancer and was told that he only had a year to live. Who knew for certain that this is all he had left of life? How could someone who did not even know him make this callow prediction to him and expect him not to respond with anger? The expression of anger is the second stage of the Kubler-Ross theory and in the case of my father, he bypassed the first stage of Kubler-Ross's theory altogether. My father had one moment of denial after he expressed his anger by saying "Why me?" But this in itself was not denial but an exclamation of grief. There was no bargaining for my dad. He did not say that he would give his eye teeth if God would let him live out his days. He did get depressed and never entered the acceptance stage as predicted by the theory.

With respect to bargaining, I am reminded of the old Jewish grandmother who was walking her young grandson on the beach. Suddenly a giant sleeper wave rolled up on the beach and swept the young boy away. The grandmother in a frenzy started bargaining with God. She yelled out, "Oh, God, please give my grandson back to me. I will do anything. I will go and pray on a daily basis. I will be a better person. I will clean my neighbor's house. I will always tell the truth from now on." And so on and so on … Suddenly, on the next wave, the boy was washed up on the beach immediately standing next to his grandmother. The grandmother was so startled as she looked at the boy, she could only think of saying one thing to God. Looking up and clutching her grandson dearly she spoke, "God, he had a hat. Where is his hat?!"

There is always some measure of compromise in bargaining either with God or the devil; however, bargaining never turns out the way we hope it will. There is no free lunch, as the saying goes. Faith has a lot to do with people who are dying, but attitude is far more important with respect to acceptance, fighting to stay alive, or just plain dealing with the situation at hand. As American writer and clergyman Charles R. Swindoll said:

> *The longer I live, the more I realize the impact of attitude on life. Attitude, to me, is more important than facts. It is more important than the past, the education, the money, than circumstances, than failure, than successes, than what other people think or say or do. It is more important than appearance, giftedness or skill. It will make or break a company ... a church ... a home. The remarkable thing is we have a choice everyday regarding the attitude we will embrace for that day. We cannot change our past. We cannot change the fact that people will act in a certain way. We cannot change the inevitable.*
>
> *The only thing we can do is play on the one string we have, and that is our attitude... I am convinced that life is 10 percent what happens to me and 90 percent of how I react to it. And so it is with you ... we are in charge of our Attitudes.*

In hindsight, looking back some quarter of a century at my dad's process of dying, I find it rather interesting as an "involved observer" that my dad's desperation permeated the entire process. Because I only have the memory of his actions alone and not his words, I can only judge what he was feeling from a nonverbal interpretation of how he responded during the time between being told he was going to die and his actual death. I have seen this several times: others who followed suit and became tacit and lived in the silence of their own pain, not realizing that by talking it out, they could have died in peace.

My father exhibited his anger by making demands of others in the family, rejecting affection, words of encouragement, and helpful attempts at getting him to give in to his illness in order to accept what was happening. It was almost as if he wanted to punish us all for being bystanders and not compatriots with the same ailment and temperament. The closer the time came to his demise, the more he rejected us and the quieter he got. There was no closure for any of the family members and especially not for him.

In making peace with the death process for my father it was necessary to write him a letter, after the fact, with all my feelings—good and bad—about his dying and essentially abandoning each of us in the family. I felt it was important to tell my father how much I loved him and how much others loved him for what he was to them and what he did for everyone. Somehow in doing this task, I hoped that he would hear my thoughts and know that he was loved and forgiven for not telling us how he felt about us. I also wrote him these thoughts and feelings in an effort to heal myself. Ironically, for at least a year, grieving was difficult for me, and I did not cry the entire time I was involved with his death or immediately afterward.

I learned about letter writing with respect to a deceased parent or a missing spouse or loved one through a book by Harold H. Bloomfield called *Making Peace with your Parents* (Ballantine Books, 1990). From the time I read the book until the present, I have been a strong advocate of not only handling painful experiences by journaling (writing these thoughts down) but also by writing to those people who are no longer available, for one reason or another, who have ultimately impacted one's life enough to cause emotional pain.

About a year after the death of my father, I discovered that I had a patient who was dying of cancer. She was about eighty years young, and her daughter asked me to come to her home one night. I remember this woman for her principles and convictions because she at one time sat in the middle of the road preventing semitrucks and trailers, eighteen wheelers to be exact, from driving through a residential neighborhood. She sat in the middle of the street knitting in a lounge chair—immovable—thus forcing the trucks to take back roads to leave the community, rather than go through the residential part itself. She had a lot of spunk and guts!

I went to her daughter's home on request, where the old woman lay dying in a large bed. Her family was around her. There was classical music playing within the room, which was darkened, lit only by candlelight. My elderly patient was draped in soft, woolen blankets. She bid me come close, and as I bent over her she rose to kiss my forehead. She told me how much she loved me, appreciated me, and thanked me for taking such good care of her all the years she was my patient. I thanked her for being my patient, and told her how much I cared about her and respected her. This was a mutual love affair that had seen many years in the dental office but never in such personal space.

I turned around and left the house hurriedly walking to my car across the street. I put the key in the ignition, but never turned it on. The tears began to flow and flow—they continued for about an hour. I realized sometime down the line that these were tears not just for her but for my dad as well. After that, I felt as if a large weight had been taken off my shoulders. My patient's death was the complete antithesis of my father's death in reality. Her death was also the catalyst I needed to begin the grieving process for myself. We could only wish that my father would have died in peace, at home, with his family and friends by his side but it never happened that way. My father's death was a death filled with pain—physical for my dad and emotional for the family—coupled with much coldness from a hospital room filled with technology, noise, mayhem, and total depersonalization. That coldness, so to speak, was further transmitted to the cemetery as I remember the coldness of my father's body when I touched him in the coffin, the silence of the many friends and relatives who could not or would not say a word to me the entire time, and finally, to the cement headstone that so finalized the painful journey of my father into a wall of stone. As I stood there, looking at the wall, I could not help but think that some greater glory awaited my dad.

> *Do not stand at my grave and weep,*
>
> *I am not there, I do not sleep I am a thousand winds that blow,*
>
> *I am the diamond glints on snow.*
>
> *I am the sunlight on ripen grain, I am the gentle autumn's rain,*
>
> *When you awaken in the morning hush, I am the swift uplifting rush of quiet birds in circled flight,*
>
> *I am the soft star that shines at night,*
>
> *Do not stand at my grave and cry. I am not there; I did not die.*
>
> —*Mary Elizabeth Frye, American poet, "I Am Not There"*

Dr. Eric Z. Shapira, DDS, MA, MHA

THE GRIEVING PROCESS

The grieving process is highly individual, much like the experience of dying. It is a process in which the survivors of death need to either rationalize their own feelings or come to grips with reality about the person who is now leaving or gone from their lives. These are difficult times for everyone, especially children, and it is incumbent upon parents to reach out with open and honest responses, conveying to them what is happening and the necessity to grieve when loss occurs.

When my father died, I was older but still did not have the ability to grieve in a way that could take away my anxiety about the situation. I was forced to intercede as the strong son who could handle the situation, help my mother with the details of the funeral, and aid my siblings in the process of their own sorrow, all along denying my own feelings in order to maintain some order and decorum, or basic control of the situation.

The famous pediatrician, Dr. Benjamin Spock, has been quoted in an article titled "Death: Answering your Preschooler's Questions," as saying, "All healthy people of every age have some degree of fear and resentment of death. There is no way to present the matter to children that will get around this basic human attitude. But if you think of death as something to be met eventually with dignity and fortitude you'll be able to give somewhat the same feeling about it to your child."

It was unfortunate for Dr. Spock that he had to go back and examine his philosophy about dying when his own child committed suicide. His degree of resentment was probably internalized and his thinking that he was to blame for this tragedy might have caused a momentary blindness in his grieving process. This makes things very difficult with regard to starting or even completing the healing process.

Since one of the basic premises of this book is dignity, dying with dignity comes above all else. The age-old question of how do we make this come about is a difficult one. Many people do not want to be told what to do or accept aid in any way that will limit their independence. They allow pride to take precedence over the mundane aspects of functioning in everyday life. It's important to convey to those who wish to maintain their dignity while they're in the midst of the dying process a kind of reverse psychology thinking: The person who is dying will then be helping those who will eventually be left behind. The survivor will gain pleasure by enabling the dying person to stay connected in some way. This way the dying person maintains dignity throughout the dying process—playing a helpful role, making others feel at ease. For some reason, this works!

People who are chronically ill and dying, and who feel that there is little or no personal dignity left, sit back, watch, and allow others to do for them if so inclined. This action allows everyone involved to feel good. In turn, this activity sets the tone for a smooth transition to an early jump start on the grieving process by all those who will be left behind to grieve and eventually heal.

Also as part of the grieving process are the cultural customs with such things as sitting Shivah for one week for those of the Jewish faith, or the wake for Catholics and other Christians. Each of these processes involves traditions, eating, rituals, and sitting with the family to comfort them.

Los Dias de las Muertes or Days of the Dead is a Hispanic custom found south of the border and in the United States as well, encompassing death as a celebration of life. Family and friends meet and greet over the grave, hold a feast, sing and dance, and memorialize their loved ones. I had the pleasure of this experience in Oaxaca, Mexico several years ago when I visited a graveyard on Halloween night during the

Day of the Dead celebration. There was plenty of mescal, a Mexican drink about five times stronger than tequila, complete with the worm in the bottom of the bottle to give the liquor an extra kick.

I had the pleasure of digging a grave above the actual plot of one family's grandfather and placing his photos and some of his personal relics there to memorialize him. We sang songs, ate wonderful home-cooked food, and held hands. The families included me as if I were one of their own, and believe me, I felt like one of them (and that was not the mescal talking either!). All of this celebration is designed to ease the pain of dying on the survivors and to honor their ancestors. I think between the liquor, the dancing, the meal, the staying up all night to party, and the lack of sleep there is a kind of euphoria or trance state that one enters into, which elevates the psyche to a mysterious higher level of consciousness. At this point, one cannot only visualize the deceased, but one can appreciate the bond that occurs between the family and friends with respect to the person whose life is being celebrated.

Funerals are a custom we have in our lives, and even though they can be expensive, they allow us a vehicle for the acknowledgment of the death that has occurred, aiding the survivors, allowing them to reorient themselves from the shock of death and providing a recognized way to dispose of the body legally, ethically, and morally.

Grieving on all fronts is necessary in order to heal. One must allow the expression of emotions; allow oneself permission to feel, and to share these feelings with others. I always recommend that people consider taking a hot shower, which in turn relaxes the body and allows one to cry, releasing emotions necessary to help the grieving process. This process can be used for any loss. Grieving can also be done in silence using meditation techniques for relaxation and guided imagery, which allows one to visualize emotions, being in a different place or seeing the healing begin from the inside out.

Counseling is recommended for younger children who cannot cope and adults who have similar problems. Blockage of feelings, tears, and the ability to talk about how you feel in the face of despair or trauma can be limited through counseling and subsequent rejuvenation of the soul. Counseling is a safe environment for people to be able to express themselves and also to learn how to express their feelings in words. Counseling may take several or many visits before results are brought forth, but however difficult this may be, a person will have a greater ability to heal over time through this medium.

Preparation and the Legacy

People who are going to die soon can help survivors and loved ones by preparing for their death both legally and spiritually. Leaving a legacy is the ability to express one's thoughts on paper, tape, CD, or DVD. The legacy will illustrate why and how a person would like to be remembered. This process will also allow the dying person to include his or her feelings, emotions, and thoughts about who he or she really is with respect to those who will be left behind. One might think of a legacy as a leg up on being prepared for death and not being around personally to tell those whom one cares about that they were perceived in their thoughts, taking them with you in spirit.

Being ahead of the game, in a sense, means being able to prepare thoughts, information, and feelings about people you know, imparting mutual respect and love to them when you are not among them anymore. This shows forethought and caring. Moving into death without this tool leaves people wondering about where they stood in your thoughts and in your life and taps into their insecurities about whether they were important to someone they may have loved and respected or at least thought of as a good friend.

Where do we start when writing a legacy? Organize your thoughts by listing all those people who made a difference in your life. Put their names down a column or place one name at the top of each page. Then, next to their name, write the feelings and thoughts that come to mind when you think of them. Write down any events that bring a smile to your face or a tear to your eye and that made a difference in your life. When it comes time to being poetic about your life, include all these feelings, thoughts, and instances in a way that will tell people how much they meant to you or how important they were to you. This can be poetic, written in prose, or just a list of attributes that were important in your life concerning these people. Some people make a video talking about these thoughts, while others record their thoughts on tape or a CD. It really doesn't matter how the legacy is communicated, as long as one completes something which shows loved ones that they were important to you.

> *Observe the Universe: aimless specks of light in a sea of darkness; giving direction to the unknown.*
>
> *Observe death: single events in life ending in darkness; finding meaning in a microcosm of human interaction.*
>
> *Memories: Validation of explorers whose quests for purpose find the light in silent words; unlocking the darkness of their souls with the knowledge that they have made a difference.*
>
> —Eric Zane Shapira, "Our Universe"

Extremely Important Documents

How can you prepare for a death in a manner that is organized, effective, and will cause little to no hassle for family members? First, you must make sure you have a durable power of healthcare. This is a legal document that spells out how you should be treated medically, assuming that you personally have no more control over what happens to you by verbal or other means of command. If you do not want someone to pull the plug on you, or if you do want the plug pulled even when there still may be a chance that you will recover from a serious stroke, heart attack, or accident, then it is necessary for you to have this document. You can make definitive comments that will control a situation that would otherwise be out of your control. That is, you can dictate how treatment should proceed, how and when all methods of resuscitation should be abandoned, and the like in this document. The alternative is not to have this document and leave your fate in someone else's hands, leaving your family responsible for dealing with uncertainty during an already stressful time.

The power of attorney allows an immediate family member or even an unrelated person the ability to administer the legal and financial aspects of an estate after the person in question can no longer function in a rational manner to maintain the business of everyday life, including handling his or her legal or business affairs. Holding the power of attorney is a powerful position to be in and is the cause of much dissention if there are siblings who feel they deserve far more than the will suggests. This honor, if you will, should be chosen with extreme caution, foresight, and wisdom. Knowledge of how a person thinks, how they act under pressure, and how a person will respond to family dynamics is important when choosing who will represent you.

A will is an important document to have, as it allows you to dictate how personal belongings and possessions will be allocated and distributed after your death. This includes money as well as other material things. Without a will, the government will handle the distribution of funds and possessions without input from family or others who might wish to have a say in the matter. Legal battles may ensue as a result of not writing a will and the cost of this action, both monetarily and emotionally, is high and should be avoided.

There are different kinds of wills that can be used by anyone wanting to dictate how their material possessions should be distributed. A holographic will is one that is handwritten and signed and that expresses what that person would like to leave behind and to whom. Some states do not recognize holographic wills as valid, and those that do generally have stringent conditions for such a document to be deemed valid. These types of wills are not considered substitutes for a formally executed will.

I have a friend who was left a large sum of money, fifty thousand dollars, by an acquaintance of his. He was overjoyed at the fact that someone he hardly knew was giving him this gift. As he waited in exuberant anticipation for several weeks after the death of the person who was willing him the money, he received another letter stating that there was a signed addendum to the will that was brought forth by the widow, superseding and canceling the bequeathing of any money to my friend. Needless to say, he was crushed by this news. Apparently the wife, a second or third wife of the gentleman in question, had him sign the holographic addendum while he was on the verge of death and consumed with dementia, leaving everything to her. The addendum was a holographic will, and it stood up in court as such.

My friend was going to challenge this action legally but realized that he would probably be paying more in legal fees than he would have received from the will, if anything at all. This episode turned out to be a futile situation for my friend, to say the least. I think he was also lucky not to have bought that new car he dreamed about when he first thought of receiving this lump sum.

Wills can also be downloaded, online, then filled out and taken to an attorney for review and filing. There are many ways to write a will, and what one feels is best for them should be discussed with an attorney. Either way, it is better to have one then not.

A trust is another vehicle that spells out who should get what in a more exacting way with the necessary legal jargon and usually is prepared by the family attorney. Trusts usually ensure that a portion of an inheritance is tax exempt, assuming they are written to protect the inheritors. There are many different kinds of trusts and it is best to seek out an elder law attorney or a trusts and estates attorney to have one drawn up. There are revocable and irrevocable trusts that necessitate study in order to determine which one is best for a particular person. When one is handling the affairs of an elder parent who might be considering going into an assisted-living situation or a skilled nursing facility it is important to look at these trust documents and their respective duties and specifications before the parent enters a facility.

If a parent has considerable assets and needs to enter a skilled nursing facility, the parent may not qualify for payment by Medicare or Medicaid. Assets may be transferred into a trust for the family; the parent may keep his or her home and at least two thousand dollars in the bank to qualify for Medicare or Medicaid to help pay for a skilled nursing facility. The family must make sure the money and assets are transferred at least five years in advance to qualify. So know before you go, so to speak, as these things from the perspective of having to pay mega-taxes or guarantees signed by family members in light of thinking that Medicare will take care of everything, when it doesn't, are important in the end.

A spiritual will or ethical will is another document that most people don't know about. In these types of wills, people can specify what kind of service they would like, how they want people to respond and act during the funeral process, and the kind of burial they would like as well. People can even write their ceremonies for the funeral and make a recording of themselves to be played at the funeral, giving people last wishes and blessings.

Spiritual wills are sometimes accompanied by certain rituals. Some people make paper coffins and have the family and guests write messages to put in them. After this task, the small paper coffins are placed in the real coffin and buried with the deceased. Letters to the deceased can also be included as part of the healing process of the family or friends. There can be an expressed desire for a memory book with photo collages and perhaps a CD or a DVD. A journal can be made of the life history of the person that can be read at the funeral or afterward by guests. And of course, the party. Don't forget the party-on part of the death process. From the marching band to a symphony orchestra, dancing girls or guys, to babies tap-dancing—whatever one can afford or imagine can be arranged to memorialize a person who has passed away. These things are all part of the process of writing down, beforehand, what one desires during a funeral and afterward. One needs to die with no regrets.

> *I would rather be ashes than dust! I would rather that my spark should burn out in a brilliant blaze than it should be stifled by dry-rot. I would rather be a superb meteor, every atom of me in magnificent glow, than a sleepy and permanent planet. The proper function of man is to live,*

not to exist. I shall not waste my days in trying to prolong them. I shall use my time.

—Jack London, American writer, *Tales of Adventure*

Special Awareness

Death and dying involve much understanding, many needs, and a whole lot of communication. Many people who are dying need to have the process explained to them in order to limit the amount of anxiety or fear that they may encounter along the way. A near-death experience, according to Maggie Callanan, RN, a hospice nurse who wrote a book called *Final Gifts* (Bantam Books, 1997), has a special knowledge about, and sometimes control over, the process of dying.

Coming close to death can bring on all kinds of aberrations for the patient and many mysteries that need to be interpreted for the immediate family as well as getting a handle on communication with both the patient and any medical staff at hand. Death is a solemn moment, as is the process of dying. It is within the boundaries of these two events that truth is usually filleted and laid out in the open for others to observe. Repentance, guilt, sadness, joy—a flood of emotions can come bursting through the gates of many years of walled-up feelings and thoughts.

This is a time where patience, understanding, and open communication need to be put in play. Knowing that time is running out, many people wish to discuss their frailties and their wishes with others, not specifically family. Therefore, one must be prepared to handle these things and encourage people to continue to talk about their feelings in a safe environment where judgment is not a factor. Listening is a gift we can give to people at this time in their lives. Active listening will allow us to have the people we are listening to verify what they are feeling after we echo what we think they feel. Active listening, in the form of nonjudgmental paraphrasing of what others are saying, is what helps people the most, letting them know that they are being heard and cared for overall by the listener.

Grieving starts even before someone dies. It can manifest itself through anxiety, crying, loquaciousness or silence, and moving inward. It is incumbent upon those who are part of the process of dying to recognize these signs and symptoms and encourage those who are affected by the dying process to share their feelings and thoughts with others. This is where a good support group is necessary. Whether it is one made up of immediate family members, friends, or strangers going through the same process, the group allows people in the same situation to share in the process of death and dying, making the transition easier and maybe a little less painful for everyone involved.

Upon asking my mother what she got out of her support group after her husband, my father, died, her comment to me was, "The support group helped me to relax. I was able to understand what was happening to me in a better way and uncover my feelings about what had happened. I was able to make new friends who had similar experiences. We got together on a regular basis, which was most comforting, allowing me to continue to share my feelings and to heal in a quicker fashion along with my friends."

Out of the ashes rose the phoenix; my mother at age sixty began to relive life, learn new things, begin to date again, write, enjoy life on a different level, and start the process of defining herself without relating to my father in the way that she had done for over forty years. It was time for her to be herself, whoever that was. Most people will begin to find the same route to self-discovery after a spouse or a loved one dies. This does not mean that they completely forget about the loved one, not in any way, shape, or form. How could someone forget a person they lived with, loved, and played with for over forty years? That is not about to happen. The process of dying and death creates rebirth in those that remain behind. This process forces one to explore his or her inner self, combining these entities with the outer self in relation to the world, in order to determine what is right for them with respect to continued living.

Viktor Frankl, author of *Man's Search for Meaning* (Washington Square Press, 1964), spoke of the psyche of Man as being a closed system, meaning that Man needs to look at the outside world in order to find himself. The process of self-actualization relates to this phenomenon, but self-transcendence is what really happens as one looks for a higher meaning to life in the face of stress or disaster, like losing a loved one.

With respect to grieving and transcendence, I am reminded of a patient of mine who, for many years, came to my clinic for care. He drove a big Mercedes automobile and was a very fine commercial, graphic artist with a successful business. But this man was born with no legs or arms, at least as we know them to be for normal people. How could it be that this person, I'll call him Sam, did everything normal people do, but wasn't physically normal himself?

I think that Sam spent many years transcending his perceptions of what normal was and in essence came to the realization many years before that in spite of the disability, which some may say he had, he would be normal in all the aspects of the word. Sam's artwork is superb and his ability to carry on the functions of everyday life are sufficient to allow him to do things even some normal people could not do with all their limbs!

So, how does this come about? Maybe Sam's mother and father had misgivings and guilt about the way he turned out due to his mother having taken Thalidomide before he was born. This was a drug that was taken for migraine headaches before anyone ever knew that it caused severe birth defects. I am sure there was a lot of grieving for this child when he was a baby and even up until he was able to prove to others that he could do things that normal people do. He was not going to give up, nor was he going to die because of his disability. In all the years that I saw Sam and spent time with him, he never once complained or parted without the smile on his face. Other people might grieve for his loss, but he transcended time to another place in order to overcome his adversity in the face of being dead, in this case, that being someone who gave up absolutely nothing in life due to a handicap.

> *Even in the deepest sinking there is the hidden purpose of an ultimate rising. Thus it is for all men, from none is the source of light withheld unless he himself withdraws from it. Therefore the most important thing is not to despair.*
>
> —*Hasidic Saying*

Grieving can accommodate many different kinds of losses should one seek to grieve in a personal way. Personal loss constitutes not only the figurative loss of self or how we perceive others within us, but also the literal loss of self; whether that be in body parts or sense of self. Grieving is a vehicle that carries us to far-off places where we can escape our pain or it can be a platform for us to look at ourselves, our own lives allowing us to feel life as we know it and grow from the experience. Without the grief process we cannot hope to live a happy life. We will endeavor to carry pain and sorrow to the end of our days. Who says we need to punish ourselves so much that we don't experience the fullness of life because we are too downtrodden with pain, hurt, guilt, and subsequent anxiety left from our losses that we did not or could not cope with over time? Life is an individual set of experiences that one must decide how to personally interpret. Forgiveness at this juncture is not only necessary, but the vehicle personally that allows one to heal in the face of much pain and suffering.

> *I am but a single cell*
>
> *Multiplied by the thousands.*
>
> *I am but a single thought*
>
> *Changed by each moment in time*
>
> *I sing, but not out loud,*
>
> *Praises of life's gifts*
>
> *The air, the water, the food,*
>
> *The sky, the people around me, my gifts all.*
>
> *I cry, but not out loud,*
>
> *For lost souls and pieces of myself*
>
> *Friends who are no longer there,*
>
> *Family who are physically gone,*
>
> *Pets who have etched a vision in my heart,*
>
> *My gifts all.*
>
> *But now I see a vision of life ...*
>
> *A melodious chorus of notes*
>
> *that have touched my soul in someway:*
>
> *A symphony of sorts, played out*
>
> *Under the stars;*
>
> *Embracing, yet another night of*
>
> *Music that brings a smile to my face*

> *And warmth with the understanding that soon,*
> *I will be part of the song.*
>
> —Eric Zane Shapira, "I Am"

Hospice Care

Hospice has been a recognized entity for almost fifty years now. The word "hospice" takes its root from the word "hospitality," yet it can be a frightening word and thought for most due to its associations with dealing with the dying. Looking back in history, hospice found its roots in facilities or shelters providing comfort and care to sick or weary travelers on long journeys.

In Europe, monks were the caregivers, and people were kept in monasteries until they recovered enough to continue their journeys. Medical care at that time was limited, and what these specific people received was a form of palliative care. Today palliative care is fast becoming a specialty of medicine and nursing and is a precursor to actual placement in hospice care before a person dies. Special medical teams are formed to triage patients to determine the extent of their illness. Once a diagnosis is made, the patient can be sent to whatever section of the hospital or skilled nursing facility is best equipped to accommodate their needs until the end of their life.

The modern day hospice was founded in London by Dame Cicely Saunders. She was a physician in the 1960s who trained as a social worker and nurse. Several things occurred on her watch that became important aspects of hospice care. One major thing was the discovery of Brompton's cocktail, a mixture of medicines that was given as an elixir (contained alcohol) for the relief of pain. A second discovery was that of the importance of the holistic/psychological approach to the relief of emotional and spiritual suffering.

Hospice care continued to flourish and was aided by two federal programs started in 1965, the advent of Medicare and Medicaid benefits in the United States. In the 1980s and 1990s hospice was included in these federal subsidy programs. Today, these benefits consist of two ninety-day periods initially followed by an unlimited number of renewable sixty-day periods of coverage. Care is offered to those who are suffering from end-stage disease such as congestive heart failure, chronic obstructive pulmonary disease, renal failure, Parkinson's disease, late-stage Alzheimer's disease, and other illnesses that are deemed life threatening, such as cancer as long as documentation for the steady decline of the individual can be presented.

Hospice care involves the use of team dynamics and ancillary specialists including: a physician, trained volunteers, nurses, social services specialists, home-health aides, chaplains, grief support specialists, children's specialists, and whatever else it takes to assist the patient and the family through the process of dying. The hospice nurses are usually on call twenty-four hours per day, seven days a week to assist in care. In my experience, hospice care is usually called for too late by the physician. Several attempts have been made to educate the community about hospice so that they will put pressure on their physicians to call on hospice earlier. In turn, for the benefit of not only the patient but the families of patients who are also suffering. All too often hospice is called less than a week before a person dies when it could be recognized as appropriate as much as six months to a year earlier.

I had a dear friend who found out too late that he had colon cancer. This is a perfectly preventable disease if people take the time to have colonoscopies on a regular basis. My friend was a victim of supervised neglect and fear, for colon cancer ran in his family. Need I say more? By the time it was discovered, my friend had developed peritonitis (an infection of the peritoneal cavity due to a rupture in a diseased organ or the colon itself) and this allowed the disease to spread. Eventually, the disease moved to his liver and then it was only a matter of time. He suffered with treatment for about six months before he was put on hospice care and died two weeks later. I assume that he could have been placed in hospice care a lot earlier; however, it did not happen. In the end, the hospice workers were there daily, helping his wife and other family members cope with the disease and its side effects and the stress of the situation for everyone.

My friend suffered a great deal and it even became necessary to find morphine for him illegally, which would not have been necessary if people were aware of the law. A law was passed several years ago that allows a physician to prescribe morphine one time and then have it automatically renew on demand once a person is in hospice; but in this case no one knew this law existed. My friend's private physician pilfered the office stash of morphine for his patient to keep him from experiencing too much pain one night. It didn't make sense that this kind of thing had to take place.

Dying with dignity is an important aspect of hospice care and the wish of almost every person I know. Sometimes this is difficult to achieve because some people do not know the laws, the system, or the existence of hospice and what it does or provides in the face of death. Dignity is a precious commodity and needs to be savored and nurtured, both within and without the individual during his or her journey. Hospice care is a final gift we can give someone—one that will uphold their dignity as a human being in the face of depersonalization by the disease they may have and the care they may or may not ultimately receive.

> *The truth is that **there** is only one terminal dignity—love. And the story of a love is not important—what is*

important is that one is capable of love. It is perhaps the only glimpse we are permitted of eternity.

—*Helen Hayes, American actress*

Hospice care is shared love. Shared love is the expenditure of energy by many good people in the form of caring, empathy, prayer, affection, wiping someone's bottom, feeding, reading or singing, laughing, telling jokes in the face of adversity, holding another, communicating with all six senses, and holding up someone you don't even know when they can't do it for themselves, just to name a few. When the time comes, you will know that calling hospice or having your physician do it for you is the best choice to make.

Hospice care can take place at home, or in a hospital if need be, but it allows one who is dying the ability to be at home as long as possible and to die at peace in surroundings that are familiar and comfortable, making the dying process more acceptable.

If you have read the book, *Tuesdays with Morrie* (Doubleday, 1997) by Mitch Albom, or even if you haven't, this sets a fine example of a dying man at home and the love and care he received during the process, especially from a friend. My father's doctor did not call hospice, which would have allowed clergy to come in daily, around the clock nurses and home-health aides to care for him so that my mother and the rest of the immediate family would not have had to struggle so much, allowing my father the ability to stay in his home where he surely would have been more at ease and possibly accepting of what was happening to him. My entire family felt that my father's physician was insensitive and did not pay enough attention to him during this process, even though he himself was struggling with the death of his patient.

My mother, on the other hand, was forced to make a decision when my father became ill, by sending her mother, who was living in our house at the time, to an assisted-living facility. She could not take care of both my grandmother and my father concurrently. These types of choices promote guilt and much mental angst. It did not matter at this juncture that my father did not want hospice care because of his perception that it meant he was going to die. My father did not understand the ramifications of his actions then and did not comprehend the nature of his disease, having never let himself investigate what his options were in light of his blinding anger. Counseling could have helped but this is hindsight now. Whether he, like others, would have allowed himself the luxury of counseling is an unknown at this point. Hospice would have helped keep a lot of emotional pain from happening had the family known about it back then and had the ability to make choices regarding subsequent care.

> *The future is not a result of choices among alternative paths offered by the present, but a place that is created—created first in the mind and will, created next in activity. The future is not some place we are going to, but one we are creating. The paths are not to be found, but made, and the activity of making them, changes both the maker and the destination.*
>
> —*John Schaar, Professor Emeritus, UC Santa Cruz*

In reality, everyone should know about hospice and what it does. If someone does not know, then it is easy enough to find out before you need it. Even if you might think it is too late for hospice, the time is never too late for hospice and what it brings. People should not have to suffer in their final hours, and hospice makes sure that every conceivable thing that can be done to alleviate physical and emotional pain, bringing spiritual peace and harmony to the family in a time of great personal stress and grief. The knowledge that comes with hospice is imparted to each and every person affected by the dying process.

Hospice is inexpensive for the most part and is covered by insurance and Medicare. Most of the time is at a low enough cost that people can afford it should they not have insurance. Some hospices even provide free care in extreme cases. So no one should be without this modality to help in a time when an extra hand is needed to help ease the burden of death and dying on a family and on the dying individual.

What I have learned from elders who never acted their age regarding the dying, grieving part of life, is to allow myself the freedom to choose how I want to die, how I will relate to death by understanding it before I let it take me, and certainly helping those around me grieve before the final event, should I get the chance. I wish to celebrate my death as an integral part of my life and all that I have accomplished.

By doing this, I am sharing love with those around me. I am a teacher. By being a teacher, I impart love to others by giving them my teachings. Showing people my own sense of mortality is enlightening for me and hopefully for them, allowing them a greater freedom to understand their own frailness. In light of the dying process, it is important to teach others what to expect from something they may not know anything about or have fear about with respect to their own lives.

I have seen people die in the most gentle of ways in dim light, soft music, surrounded by the people they love and are loved by in peace. I have also seen death come to those in cold rooms with no recognition of others around them and the loss of love and sharing, only gloom and sadness. How wonderful it is to be able to communicate before death takes us and before we are not able to impart our love to others.

The beauty of life is, while we cannot undo what is done, we can see it, understand it, learn from it and change; so that every new moment is spent not in regret, guilt, fear or anger, but in wisdom, understanding and love.

—*Jennifer Edwards, American actress*

Chapter 9

Aging in Place

WHEN YOU DON'T FEEL LIKE MOVING ANYMORE!

The Senility Prayer
"God grant me the senility to forget
The people I never liked anyway,
The good fortune to run into the ones that I do,
And the eyesight to tell the difference."

—Unknown Author

I had an old nun for a patient once, Sister "Mary What's-Her-Name." She was in a quandary about whether to get out of the church at her age (seventies) and enjoy some of the life that she had not been able to partake of for most of her cloistered life. In her many hours of silent meditation one weekend, while at the monastery, she came to some conclusions for herself, one of which she etched on a piece of clay for me to hang up in my office. The pottery shard succinctly states, "When you are through changing, you're through!" How wonderful I thought as I read it, not thinking that Sister Mary was going to be changing what's-her-name right in front of my eyes to something else!

She had made a decision to leave the church after all these years and try to learn to be someone else, someone she had longed to be for over fifty years. It was time for change but it was risky, dangerous, frightening, exciting, wondrous, ostentatious, exploratory, time consuming, energy provoking, and above all a mystery for Mary all at the same time. What consternation and confusion this created for her. What chaos!

Taking a chance on a new life after seventy years is what bravery and willpower are all about (or maybe a little foolishness as well). Sister Mary was going from a life of comfort, so to speak, to a life of unknown circumstances. I thought it would be fun for Mary to learn about the world she never knew and was about to enter.

Many people who reach this age don't feel inclined to work or spend any effort moving or improving. "Retirement for me," one person might have said, "is the time of life when I have earned the right to do what I want: absolutely nothing!" But of all the hundreds of people over the age of sixty-five that I have met, very few have said these words, and of those few, most of them have found it virtually impossible to do "absolutely nothing" without going stark, raving mad.

> *"The Self desires only what is real, thinks nothing but what is true. Here people do what they are told, becoming dependent on their country, or their piece of land, or the desires of another, so their desires are not fulfilled and their works come to nothing, both in this world and in the next. Those who depart from this world without knowing who they are or what they truly desire have no freedom here or hereafter. But those who leave here knowing who they are*

and what they truly desire have freedom everywhere, both in this world and in the next."

—Eknath Easwaran, *The Upanishads*

Little do we know what the future holds for any of us. We do know that life has taken on the ability to be extended for most of us past the historical limits to longevity in past centuries. Many people have found that life is there to live, having lived life to its fullest each day. Against all odds and the wishes of the Surgeon General for one, many people continue to disobey the dictates of experts who admonish them to exercise regularly, find new interests, learn new skills, stay social, stretch their limits, and dance at least three times a week for at least 30 minutes to stave off the rigors of Alzheimer's disease.

We know that companies are laying off the older workers in order to save money and at the same time hiring them back as consultants without benefits. These corporations realize the wealth of knowledge and information that this cohort of people carries with it and how wasteful it would be to let them retire into oblivion. More people over the age of sixty-five are now finding new ways to reinvent themselves: learning a new career, discovering the joy of traveling, finding a new mate, changing the way their lives used to be, and looking for more positive and productive ways to function and live. On the other hand, many people desire to retire to a place of comfort, play golf, and eat fine food on a daily basis, if they can afford this lifestyle. But I don't see this happening to too many people in our society today. Most people want to and have to continue some kind of work and are looking for jobs that allow them to have cherished benefits, which help offset the hardships of our economy and life in general.

In reading the Senility Prayer, I have to laugh because at the beginning of this book I asked the question about how to make peace with the aging process. Overlooking it altogether would be a good thing, even if having poor eyesight was not a factor in the equation. However, coming to grips with who we are, why we are here, what we want out of life, what we should contribute to life, how we can help other people in the world we live in, and how we have some fun doing it can be what aging in place is all about. How can someone sit idly by and be satisfied watching TV for approximately seven hours a day, seven days a week (the national average for people over sixty-five)?

If you look at the prefrontal cortex of the brain by scanning it while watching TV, there is absolutely nothing going on—no activity whatsoever. But if you take that same person and put a crossword or Sudoku puzzle in front of him or her, have them read a book out loud, or ask them to solve a math problem, then do a scan of their brains—incredibly enough, their brain lights up like a neon sign on Broadway, in all pretty colors of red, green, and orange as the chemicals pulse through the nervous tissue of the brain similar to a rushing river moving on toward the sea. The brain is being stimulated to work, which allows the cells to function, living longer and staying younger longer. Doing nothing impedes one's ability to function properly, decreases cell life and brainpower, and allows specific chemicals in our bodies to start the process of deterioration.

A ninety-three-year-young client of mine, whom I counseled for over three years, was a very active man. When I went to his house most of the time I didn't find him where he said he would be. He told me to always go around the back of the house and he would be waiting for me, sitting in a lounge chair. One of the last times I saw him, I came around the corner of the back of the house and instead of seeing him on a lounge chair, I found him on the roof of his garage cleaning off the leaves! How the heck did he get up there?, I wondered. He would scream at me that he would be right down, but I had to laugh because at ninety-three, I knew it would be more than a few minutes before I saw him again. Factoring gravity into the equation, I would have to say that he got down a lot faster than I expected though and was not even out of breath.

Gene had cancer at the time but no one knew it, not even me. He carried on his daily routine, played the trumpet weekly in an "old boys" band and took his elderly ninety-six-year-old wife to the movies. He read books in English and in French each day. I remember he recalled his experience in detail at Pearl Harbor as the Japanese flew their planes directly above his head on December 7, 1941. I was transfixed by each word, visualizing the event, even to the point of seeing the same eyes of the Japanese pilots as they waved at him on a bluff over Diamond Head. He suddenly broke the train of concentration by changing the conversation to building a new fence alongside his house to keep the neighbor's animals from getting into his garden.

Gene was somewhat of an enigma to me because his wife said that he did not want to talk with me when I first started counseling her, but later on found that he could not keep from coming over when I was done counseling her to tell me his past and present history. He was a fascinating individual, and I loved every minute of my time with Gene. I think I lost part of myself when he died, for I lived those stories he told and hoped to be like him in some ways if I had the luck and good fortune to live as long as he did. Gene seemed never to stop doing something physical or mental. Gene had the mind of a young man at the age of ninety-four when he died peacefully.

How is it then that the antithesis of my client, Gene, can be found in those people who wish to stagnate in the time they have left? People who are not contributing their knowledge and experience to others who might otherwise need these same resources, appreciate the gifts, and learn to live life each day to its fullest, either accepting these things from others or by giving their own gifts. There are those who can and do, and then there are those who can and don't. I think it is human nature mixed in with a little genetics that makes this exchange possible. Attitude comes into play, as it is necessary to maintain a positive attitude in order to continue being active in one's older years.

A ninety-eight-year-young client of mine works in the garden daily to grow her own food and sews or crochets nightly, making sweaters and booties for the neighbors and relatives. She says she has lived a full life and is ready to go when God takes her, but she never stops doing things for herself and other people. Her acceptance of her age, her place in life, and her abilities to do things are what get her through each day. Yes, she has help with the chores and someone dedicated to drive her places when she needs it, but all in all, my client is very self-sufficient.

Another client of mine, who is ninety-four years young, similarly sews and reads, teaches her grandchildren, and takes long walks with the family dogs on a daily basis. She lives with her daughter and her daughter's family. When I was counseling her, she told me stories of her days in New Jersey, working in a clothing factory. She used to make the John Wayne's personal clothing and mail it to him. She spends her alone time reading for herself and sewing small pillows, quilts, and sachets to give to other people. She is most fastidious and self-sufficient but pines away thinking about all the friends she has who are not.

What is different about these specific types of older people that enables them to reach old age and yet keep their mental acuity, their sense of humor, and cognitive awareness levels of that of younger people, thus allowing them independence? What is the common thread that brings them forth into each day with such fervor and a zest for living? Does anyone really know the answers to these questions? I am not sure. Maybe it is the fact that they have lived long and productive, happy lives. You can come to your own conclusions.

I know when I told various people that I was writing this book about aging and dignity fitting into the scheme of things, they would ask, "What do you know about aging at your age?" I know that without dignity, people have nothing. Without a sense of humor and pride, people have nothing. I know that without knowledge and a zest to continue learning, people have nothing. I know that without a sense of humanity and forgiveness, people have nothing. I know that without physical and mental health, people have nothing. I know by watching other people, who have preceded me, about getting older and still enjoying life. I know because I have seen and known others who have died at a young age, not yet reaching that pivotal point in their lives where they could look back and pat themselves on the back, giving themselves kudos for a life worth living. I know because I want to enjoy each day, savor it, milk it, hold it, caress it, and nurture it until I have extracted every bit of whatever I can get out of it or put into it before letting go.

Life is too precious to waste the time we are given as it is a gift, since I feel we rent our space. It is, then, important to make the best of our time, fulfilling our prescribed duties whether they are our work, our play, good deeds, or a combination thereof on a daily basis. In essence, what we do with our time is the rent we pay for the space we occupy.

Are you one of the lucky ones who realizes your potential? Staying in place only amplifies the need to move toward a life that is rewarding and appreciated, not taken for granted. Too often we take our lives for granted, our loved ones for granted, our families for granted, and only contact our friends when we need something. Just because the circle of people we know is near and around us does not mean that we should not make contact routinely. In order to appreciate and cultivate these relationships one needs to look at them as the sautéing of a fine dish for a gourmet meal: stir in the ingredients of love, add a few pinches of special spice of life, pour a little fine wine for steeping and mellowing out, a dash of some special quality herbs for a unique flavor, making the dish elegant and different from any you have ever had, taking tender care not to overcook the mixture. Finally, add a dash of appreciation and attention for which you dip your finger in the mix for a quick taste to make sure it all works well before serving it up. Relationships in our lives are like this recipe: special, one of a kind, chosen, specially prepared with zest and gusto, and appreciated. One should know that taking things for granted will stifle the relationship as well as the meal. They both take work.

Rule a kingdom as though you were cooking a small fish— don't overdo it.

—Lao Tzu

Human Nature Takes Its Course

It is human nature to be curious about things. This in itself is a stimulant for the nidus that brings on growth through learning about the world around us. One must show an interest in things in order to learn what that something is all about and how useful it can become to anyone who may use it. Prehistoric man only evolved through curiosity and learning about those things that made his or her life easier, therefore increasing his ability to survive the hardships life had to offer. Since our society today is one which carries with it the technology and industry to make our lives much easier in most ways, many of us do not avail ourselves of learning new things to make our lives better or more rewarding, only to increase the longevity, the good health, and the increased wealth we could have on top of all the other luxuries life has to offer.

A New Wrinkle

> *The man who works need never be a problem to anyone. Opportunities multiply as they are seized; they die when neglected. Life is a long line of opportunities. Wealth is not in making money, but in making the man while he is making money. Production, not destruction, leads to success.*
>
> —*John Wicker, Lawyer*

What gives the human being the drive to stay alive, to increase longevity, to endure, to continue to thrive in a hostile world? Maybe it is that we are all hard-wired to survive anyway by the basic chemistry, which we all possess as humans. Each of us, in our own right, seems to push the limits, but only to a point. Many give up early and die prematurely. Some people try and then know when it is their time to stop trying. Dying people I have spoken to seem to know for the most part when it is his or her time to let go. They fight and fight and try to hold on for those that are left behind, but inevitably, the will to continue living wanes, giving way to the desire for a better place.

A funny thing to think about here is a better life after death. A young man was asked by his boss if he believed in life after death, to which he replied, "Yes." His boss said, "Well, good. After you took off for your grandmother's funeral yesterday, she stopped in to see you!"

Is it our wish that people die early and not suffer? When is it time to acknowledge enough of living, and become dust, rising again as someone else? Many people I have spoken to in the past seem to relish the idea of coming back as another being or entity. All Buddhists believe in reincarnation, going back to the earth from whence they came. Aging in place may force one to look at the options available in the time one has left. An eighty-one-years-young new friend of mine has stated, "aging is for sissies!" There is no moss growing under her backside.

On the other hand, an eighty-plus-year-old man that I am acquainted with does nothing in his retirement to stimulate his mind or body. He sits most of the day in front of the TV, glued to his favorite programs. He does little socializing and has admitted to me that he has done everything he wanted to do, loved the only woman he will ever allow himself to love, and now is ready to die, which he has recently accomplished. Apparently, he had no hope for anything else in his life. He did not extend himself to teach others what he knew or to surround himself with things that would have increased his mental acuity or physical ability. So what did he gain by all of this? Peace of mind? I am not sure; however, I realize that there was an underutilized good human being here.

This gentleman had the ability to choose to be different but did not. How could he have been different one may ask? He could have donated his time to helping others. He did not. He could have learned a new language and taken a trip to the country of its origin. He did not. He could have taught a young person to read. He did not. He could have chosen to love someone again. He did not. Here, all life is a matter of choice. This gentleman even maintained a state of non-responsibility for his choices, as he just existed in time and space. What meaning is there in this? Is this how to make peace with the aging process by aging in place? I think not. But for some people I think that it is an alternative to really living life because there is no desire for self-improvement or the helping of others to improve.

Wisdom is a life that knows it is living.

—*Moravian prayer book*

Wisdom in this context is the experience and the knowledge to know that one is making a difference with his or her life with respect to the rest of society. Just as the Serenity Prayer indicates, "God grant me the serenity to accept the things I cannot change; courage to change the things I can, and the wisdom to know the difference" one must understand that whatever action results from either one's activity or inactivity, it is a reaction to understanding how one's life affects the environment that he or she inhabits. The gentleman in question may have thought that he had plenty of serenity, but in reality he lived a life of denial based on possible past guilt, anger, and inner anguish, maybe as a result of depression, which no one had informed him about possibly and probably no one would have given him this information because of the risk of being chided. Would it matter anyway? I think not in this situation.

I cite this personal experience of someone most of you reading this book would probably not want to follow as an example; however, there are plenty of people in the world of this same ilk. It is a sad state of affairs when aging comes to this kind of end. Jack London stated in his epitaph, "I would rather go out a burning meteor than a glowing ember …" He was emphatic about living each moment of each day and was creative until the end, even though he partied a little too hard, which finally did him in.

> *I bought a dog the other day … I named him Stay. It's fun to call him …. "Come here, Stay! Come here, Stay!" He went insane. Now he just ignores me and keeps typing.*
>
> —*Steven Wright, American comedian*

Humor breaks tension, and so the aforementioned quote. Recognizing one's frailties can be upsetting for some, and having misgivings about not doing things that might have made a difference to others as well as oneself can be hard to swallow. Look at all the old people sitting on street corners, braving the elements, who have possibly chosen a life of abandonment due to various reasons, including insanity. Looking at those elders who volunteer to help other people and to make this a better place to live, one can see an entirely different kind of aging in place. Aging in place for them does not mean sitting around on their *tushies* doing nothing! It means making a difference to someone else and in doing so, bringing joy to themselves. This is the essence of living life to its fullest and living longer—doing for others. It all comes down to making choices.

THE BUTTERFLY

Mariposa in Spanish, *butterfly* in English: an insect that is able to change from one form to another over time. The caterpillar does all the work, but the end result gets all the glory here. Wrapping itself in a fine silken robe, the caterpillar sleeps until the mysterious chrysalis squirms: a small worm inside this flexible façade fights to free itself into the outside world. Little does it understand the meaning of its struggle or its abilities to free itself.

I would like to repeat a story that was told to me, since it is worth repeating, of how a young man found a squirming chrysalis and cut it open to let out the beautiful butterfly, only to return the following day to find it dead on the ground below. The moral of the story is that the struggle of the beautiful butterfly is one that we all must make. Having been freed before it was ready to emerge, the butterfly's muscles for flight had not developed; hence, it could not fly. Without flight, the insect could not feed itself and died prematurely.

People of any age, but especially the elderly, have continued the fight in order to survive the rigors of life—fighting, in the sense that life goes on and you must be your own advocate for survival, learning each day what is necessary to strengthen the muscles of tenacity in order to thrive yet for another day. Here the brain must be challenged, for the brain is like a child that needs to learn new and different ways of doing things to stimulate it. Our elders must try and do things in different ways, challenging themselves and their brains to function at a maximum level as they age.

> *Happiness is a butterfly, which when pursued, is always just beyond your grasp, but which, if you will sit down quietly, may alight upon you.*
>
> *—Nathaniel Hawthorne, American writer*

Ultimate happiness, then, should be an entity that you not only contemplate but also make happen, even if it means sitting quietly for a moment to allow it to sink in. We sometimes don't know what we have because we are too busy complaining about our hardships or about what others have that we don't have. I think we just need to sit down and assess what we have for a moment. We need to do this for perspective's sake. Appreciating our self-worth and enjoying our lot in life allows us all to put things into perspective. If you think your life needs changing, then plan for change and do it! The struggle will continue until all of us leave the planet in some way. Until then, make the most of what you have and learn to make a difference to others by sharing your gifts.

I am reminded of a W. C. Fields quote at this juncture, "A dead fish can float downstream, but a live fish can swim upstream." An inane thought perhaps, but not really. It takes cognizance of life and knowledge of self in order to be able to fight whatever it is that is keeping us from moving ahead … swimming upstream in essence against the flow. Be a salmon: instinctual, strong, vigilant, persistent, engrossed, forward-directed, and totally alive! Do this just for the halibut!

What I learned from older people who never acted their age in this context is that most of them don't really think they are old. The love of life, the quest for newness, the challenges of the day, the new beginnings at dawn each day and the anticipation of the sunset bringing peace and a time for reflection are most cherished by our elders. Helping others and having younger friends is also a benefit as well as doing something constructive each day, which is also a part of the secret of not only getting through the day, but living longer, loving life and staying youthful.

> *Human happiness and human satisfaction must ultimately come from within oneself. It is wrong to expect some final satisfaction to come from money or from a computer. Do not dwell in the past; do not dream of the future, concentrate the mind on the present moment.*
>
> *—His Holiness the Dalai Lama*

Chapter 10

The Sequel

HAVE DIGNITY, WILL FIND HAPPINESS

Look to this day for yesterday is but a dream and tomorrow is only a vision,

But today, well lived, Makes every yesterday a dream of happiness

and every tomorrow a vision of hope.
Look well, therefore, to this day.

—*Sanskrit Proverb*

Being happy is a state of mind—one that is mostly fleeting and has conditions put upon it at times. There are so many different levels of happiness that it is almost impossible to define these states in a tangible way. Being happy is a feeling. We can appear happy by showing our smiles, but in reality we may not be happy. We can disguise happiness with a sad face as well. So the many facets of happiness may challenge us to look deep down inside ourselves in order to understand the nature of our happiness and how it came to be. Being happy and the state of happiness may be two entirely different conditions that need to be defined in order to determine the value we place on things before us in life. For most people, perception is their reality, which I think sometimes distorts what the real meaning is for the state of happiness and being happy.

I have found that the state of happiness may emanate from some kind of pleasure. Pleasure can be found in many things and in many ways. When I used to run half marathons, I knew that I was happy for several reasons: For one, I could run. Secondly, I knew that endorphins in my brain would kick in and tickle the pleasure center in my brain, thus making me feel happier, and lastly, having this chemical happiness allowed me to be in a continued state of happiness, overcoming the pain of running itself..

Cause and effect here was everything. Today, I find reading a good book, eating a great meal, having some quiet time to meditate, painting watercolors or sculpting, and walking in the sea air, either alone or with family and friends, a pleasure; all bringing me happiness. Chemicals, precipitated by some act, are responsible for the state of happiness, which in turn affect one's attitude about life. This physical state is not prolonged unless we continue to do whatever it is that stimulates our chemicals to continue flowing, such as eating your favorite chocolate pie, giving or getting a hug, having sex, walking and talking with a loved or cherished one, or solving Sudoku puzzles that all along you thought you couldn't do. All of these things allow one to feel happy because our brains are stimulated, producing endorphins as well as other chemicals that increase the body's ability to feel good.

The mental satisfaction one experiences from achieving something difficult can start the process of emotional energizement, subsequently allowing us to feel happy. The opposite happens, too, when we experience something negative, finding ourselves propelled toward becoming depressed. Here, chemicals other than endorphins work the opposite end of the spectrum to make us depressed and flood our gray matter with a whole lot of other emotions that can make things cloudy or foggy-minded.

Those individuals who always seem happy make it happen; I am convinced of that. I know people who wake up happy because they seem to program their dreams to give them pleasure! Funny, but it works. Being happy with oneself is a key ingredient to long life. The more we take pleasure in who we are and what we do, what we can accomplish on a daily basis, the longer we are likely to live. Being creative around this state of happiness will bring about changes in our abilities to do things. Being creative in the sense that you can do things to help others, find new interests, work with your mind and hands to create art or anything useful, such as: doing needlepoint; making quilts; cooking; volunteering at the local USO, Senior Center, Adult Day Health Center, Project Read, school district; or any other myriad of things which can impart your gifts to other's brings happiness to yourself as well as those who might appreciate the help. Feeling good about what we do in life allows us to be happy.

One of my mottos is "we don't know what gifts we have until we give them away." Serving as well as showing empathy and concern for others and making our environment a better place to live brings happiness to others.

I once went to Loch Ness in Scotland and visited a little pub there, where everyone at the bar had sworn to have seen the monster. The people in the pub were all happy and filled with a sense of wonder ... and beer! But finding Happyness (as compared to Lochness) for most of us doesn't take alcohol or a mythical creature. Finding happiness means making an opportunity or taking an opportunity to be happy.

> *If you want happiness for an hour—take a nap. If you want happiness for a day—go fishing. If you want happiness for a month—get married. If you want happiness for a year—inherit a fortune. If you want happiness for a lifetime—help someone else.*
>
> —*Chinese Proverb*

Discovering Dignity

Finding, recognizing, and possessing dignity are three keys to living a happier life. In helping others you will certainly discover inner happiness and contentment based on the power of your gifts. There has never been a day that I have not felt this emotion or failed to share my gifts with someone. Dignity defines the person who owns it, carrying with it the ability to be independent, pensive, coherent, helpful, sensitive, and forward-thinking with the ability to maintain a humanitarian attitude about life. Holding yourself in high regard is a feat that comes with meeting the demands of growing older. This mission is accompanied by possessing wisdom and abilities that can be shared with the knowledge of life you have gained with others, as well as your excellence in attitude and daily outlook. People who have a good outlook on life usually do well being their own person. Many people find that being alone impedes their abilities to be happy and supplies them with a gloomy outlook on life, leading to depression.

Most people do not like nor choose to be alone. I know other people who love their personal freedom and sense of independence by being alone. I also know of those on the opposite end of the spectrum who fear being alone. I look at this phenomenon as a fetus, alone in a dark sea of life, floating peacefully and frozen in time, squirming at times to get comfortable, only attached to the outside world by a thin cord carrying its life force and nutriments.

Akin to this is the state of becoming older, whereby elders wander in a sea of loneliness, called society, floating to and from things that bring them pleasure; this action leading to some fleeting happiness and hopefully, a sense of purpose in life. Periodically, we find ourselves stopping for rest and some support from a few acquaintances or loved ones, in order to rejuvenate the spirit in us for supporting the tireless efforts to continue the quest. However, what is it that we seek?

One of my favorite quotes comes from the British author, Jeanette Winterson, from her book, *Oranges Are Not The Only Fruit* (Pandora Press, 1985), who says, The secret of the world is this: the world is entirely circular and you will go round and round endlessly, never finding what you want, unless you have found what you really want inside yourself. When you follow a star you know you will never reach that star; rather it will guide you to where you want to go. It's a reference point, not an end in itself, even though you seem to be following it. So it is with the world. It will only ever lead you back to yourself. The end of all your exploring will be to cease from exploration and know the place for the first time. (Quote used with direct permission from the author).

Introspection, then, is an important tool that we can use to decipher inner wants and desires toward the goal of achieving both happiness and dignity. Finding yourself and knowing what you want from life is probably the most important single thing you can ever discover and learn for yourself. Albert Einstein spoke of an important facet regarding being alone and knowing that this particular status is acceptable with respect to one's adventures toward finding strength, beauty, compassion, and the need for awareness of self. In an interview with Einstein in the *New York Post*, November 28, 1972, he is quoted as having said,

A human being is a part of the whole, called by us the "universe," a part limited in time and space. He experiences himself, his thoughts and feelings, as something separate from the rest—a kind of optical delusion of his consciousness. This delusion is a kind of prison for us, restricting us to our personal desires and to affection for a few persons nearest to us. Our task must be to free ourselves from this prison by widening our circle of compassion to embrace all living creatures and the whole of nature in its beauty. Nobody is able to achieve this completely, but the striving for such achievement is in itself a part of the liberation and a foundation for inner security.

Many people I have counseled now and in the past have been locked into themselves and an environment so small that outside reality did not exist for them, only perceived awareness that reality was the world within their own boundaries. Too often we find ourselves stifled by this same kind of scenario: limiting our potential to be happy; inhibiting our ability to find love, not understanding the importance of having dignity, disengaging from learning new things, not trying to understand the world we live in, truly knowing ourselves.

Having these capacities would elevate our status to one of happiness and having a position of dignity. It would not necessarily keep us from being alone. Being alone is a choice one makes and can easily be changed consciously, should you desire to surround yourself with other people and an agenda of activities.

I had a client not too long ago who suffered from severe chronic obstructive pulmonary disease, diabetes, and obesity (he was over three hundred pounds). He was confined to a wheelchair style scooter, sharing his time between this scooter and a large easy chair that would tip back and forth, making it easier for him to get in and out of the chair when he so desired. He had lost most of his friends due to his isolation, and his wife was depressed because she felt alone, having the onerous chore of caring for her husband.

After many weeks of counseling her, I felt that she put herself in a bind by eliminating her friends and a special art group she went to weekly for years, in order to be with her husband. He, on the other hand, barked orders at her all day long to bring him books, food, writing paper, and memorabilia such as scrapbooks and photos of old friends he used to work with to keep him occupied. He very much wanted to see people, especially his old friends, but his wife found it both difficult to take him anywhere, due to his size, and very expensive due to the methods necessary to transport him as a result of having to reserve and pay for a special ambulance to get him anywhere. They had limited means. I found myself constantly making suggestions to her about getting a caregiver, going back to her art group once a week, and giving herself permission for a respite.

Her husband was all for it, but she was ruled by guilt not to do so. He was at a point where his dignity was nil, and he did not care about too many things. He was ready to die or be placed in a facility and left alone. The wife had let her dignity falter because she became a victim in the process of choosing to take care of her husband and not herself. This example shows how choice plays a role in one's happiness and dignity. Failing to make the right choices, we sometimes impede our abilities to function in a healthy way. Allowing oneself to be ruled by guilt creates further anxiety and paralyzes its victims, thereby leaving them inactive and powerless.

Your beliefs become your thoughts. Your thoughts become your words. Your words become your actions. Your actions

> *become your habits. Your habits become your values. Your values become your destiny.*
>
> —*Mahatma Gandhi, Spiritual leader*

My job as a counselor is to help remove the obstacles from my clients' state of mind, allowing them the freedom to arrive at their own conclusions. In doing so, my clients are able to make choices that help lighten their load and in turn, keep them on a path that is right for them. Being allowed to be independent is what gives a person a leg up on having dignity. Having dignity means being independent, self-sufficient, and able to solve one's own problems (with maybe a little coaching on the side).

I truly believe in destiny and that things do happen for a reason, but sometimes one must nudge a little to get people to make decisions that will affect their destiny and allow them the necessary freedom and inner strength to break out of their molds. One cannot do this part until he or she is ready and feels strong enough to follow through on the decision that needs to be made. Many people are too afraid of the consequences or of failing, and so postpone making the final decision. In reality, those people who are too complacent in their own misery may never change, because they see too much of an advantage to remaining alone and underserved.

What does it mean to be a victim? To be a victim is to give up your mojo, your power of control over self. Many people who are used to being saved or having someone else make decisions for them so that they do not have to be responsible for anything, are the ones who end up as victims. These are self-victimized people who wish to be taken care of for as long as possible. These people usually have low self-esteem and may be chronically depressed as well. The psychological state that is maintained here is called an "attachment disorder." People of this ilk want to depend on others to take care of them. They become helpless and give up their rights and their dignity and fool themselves into thinking that this is what will bring them ultimate happiness; yet in reality, they suffer silently. Lost in the darkness of their own ignorance and inability to make decisions for themselves, these people fear the unknown and taking that one giant step toward becoming self-sufficient.

> *When you come to the end of everything you know and are faced with the darkness of the unknown, Faith is knowing one of two things will happen. Either there will be something solid for you to stand on, or you will be taught how to fly.*
>
> —*Edward Teller, Physicist*

Faith in oneself is what is missing from the equation of the person who is unsure of themselves, for one reason or another. Dignity is what is lost and happiness is non-existent. How can a person of this ilk survive on his or her own power? Counseling is needed to unclutter the past, which has created specific challenges for this cohort in being able to see that they need to make the changes in their lives that they hope others will do for them.

In the long run, these people will be much better off if they learn to become self-sufficient. As these people learn to do for others, they will gain back self-esteem, dignity, and ultimately, happiness. Many elders who find themselves alone in later life not only have this type of problem, but they tend to seek out attachments to both people and possessions, becoming obsessive about their lives in general. This is a difficult condition to cope with for family and friends, who may feel put-upon in many ways and tired of being taken for granted and leaned on in some respects.

I know an older woman in her eighties who tries to ingratiate herself to everyone she meets. At first, she invites people over to her home for a meal and an evening of fun. When people feel it is time to leave, she continues trying to keep them occupied by showing them her photo album, singing songs, telling innumerable jokes, or making them more food. On a second visit of this sort, you may be one of the lucky people Gladys (not her real name) enlists to help clean out her garage, which is an all-day affair. But then, of course, you will be asked to stay for a meal, forced to listen to more jokes, join in singing, asked to eat numerous desserts, and finally, finding yourself babbling, trying to make enough excuses that will allow you the privilege of leaving without any altercation. Needless to say, these things get old after a while.

Then, after a few days go by, you might receive a call or better yet, Gladys may show up on your doorstep to see what you are doing. At this point, you want to slam the door, but not wanting to be rude, you invite Gladys into your home, and she ends up staying for dinner. Now, you might as well offer her a bed for the night because getting her to leave is almost impossible! Close to midnight, somebody yells that Gladys's car is being towed down the street, complete with her dogs inside. Once she is out of the house, all the lights are immediately turned off leaving no sign of life left on the planet … need I say more. Make sure you don't answer the phone for the next several days as well.

Gladys is a lonely person. Even though she pushes herself on others, she has a job; she has a house full of pets (about seven dogs that go everywhere with her), and she has a house full of tasks she has not yet completed. She may be lonely, but Gladys is a busy person. I think the reason she has not completed most of her projects is because she is running around trying to attach herself to whoever will give her an ear or some kind of sympathy. Gladys is a prime example of someone with an attachment disorder extraordinaire. People like Gladys usually have been married numerous times because of their need to be with someone who can take care of them. Once the husband gets the full scope of who he has married, at this point it is all over—a new ballgame with scoreless innings, so to speak.

On the other hand, an older man with this type of challenge will stay put in his home or apartment; usually because a man is not as much of a social animal as a woman. Men who have attachment problems tend to be loners; even though they have an extreme need to be with someone, they don't know how. The dichotomy here is quite disconcerting because of the polar opposite desire to be with someone and the condition that exists keeping them solo. Statistically, there is a very high suicide rate among older men who live alone and suffer from this type of problem. Getting these people out of the house is imperative to their survival in the long run, and counseling is in order to help them overcome this condition.

Recently, I had the occasion to work with a client who was in his mid-eighties. He is depressed, bipolar, and occasionally suicidal. He has cognitive decline and loss of memory. He lives alone and has lived alone most of his older life. He says he needs no one, but in reality he needs anyone who can help him. This is a prime example of what I have been talking about with respect to a loner who needs others to help him function and survive. If this person is left alone, he will barely eat and sometimes he will not remember to eat at all. He forgets what he needs to do and where he needs to go. He has trouble doing his books, paying his bills, and remembering how to use the cell phone and TV changer. This is a person who needs either a room in a facility where he will be helped to take care of himself or a caregiver 24/7. The situation is difficult, frustrating and somewhat unsolvable. Everything I have done or that his family has tried to do to help him is undone by others who have taken him away from any help and placed him back in his own environment, alone and without help. This is a no-win situation. No wonder he wants to die!

Maintaining Happiness

So, "If you want to be happy for the rest of your life, make an ugly woman your wife" as the old song goes. This way one can be assured that no one else will want her and she will stay with you forever. I am sure this works in reverse, for women too. Is that all there is, you may ask? Today many people avail themselves of opportunities such as taking many vacations, having a second home, having lots of toys, and diving into plastic surgery to change the perceived ugliness of aging or some other perceived imperfection. Plastic surgery procedures are up over 2000 percent in the past two years! We live in a society that is visually oriented and self-aggrandizing. People, mainly the baby boomers, require immediate satisfaction and results. We expect the best and want it all now. This is the wealthiest and most technologically savvy cohort of individuals our society has ever known and many people in this group can afford to buy, for the most part, anything they want, any time they want it. However, in light of the recent financial crisis things may have been scaled down a bit with respect to excessive spending on luxuries.

Maintaining one's happiness in a time of life which is evolving is a difficult thing. I am sure most people have heard the saying "money can't buy happiness," but, it's way ahead of whatever is in second place. There are no two ways about it; one can't get by too well without financial security in this world we live in. Let's accept the fact that you need to be prepared for growing older with a nest egg and enough capital to get you through hard times and changes in lifestyle. Today, having three hundred thousand dollars doesn't do it for retirement, and how many of us have that much money? With the onset of the recent financial crisis, most all of us have lost a good chunk of our nest egg. People who were retired or wanted to retire can't. Where is the happiness in this fact?

One might compare happiness to eating an ice cream sundae either by taste-testing one teaspoon at a time, savoring each morsel, or shoving the entire sundae down in two gulps. In the case of the latter, one may not be able to discern the fine taste of each ingredient by itself and how each entity melds with the others to give it maximum enjoyment and taste. This orgasmic experience allows one to experience immediate happiness which lasts for at least ten to fifteen minutes. Some might think it's better than sex, and for some it is! I find happiness fleeting and have learned to accept it in small doses rather than in big gobs at one sitting.

Happiness is all the craze these days with people looking for it high and low, near and far, but I think people need to realize that happiness will inevitably find you if you are receptive to it. Happiness will increase one's ability to stay healthy, improve one's thought processes, inspire the outpouring of more creative juices, improve earning capacity, and improve one's self-esteem as well as even escalating one's lovemaking abilities.

Many books on happiness or being happy have been written lately because this is similar to the yearning of Ponce de Leon's quest for the Fountain of Youth, coupled with people trying to locate this place, figuratively, for years. Since we live in a fast-paced society, one filled with stress and demands on an ongoing basis, people need to be able to have good coping skills in order to defend themselves from the attack of society on one's personal space.

I am reminded of my ex-wife once in a while when I think of being happy. Interesting switch of thought here ... she was not a happy person when I knew her. I think her memory conjures up a picture of an unhappy time in my life. I remember coming home one day and finding a note that read, "Remember the happy times," finding her gone, out of my life forever. I had mixed emotions and did not know whether to laugh out loud or cry. I think I did a little of both because for one, I could not remember too many happy times with her. Secondly, I was relieved that she had left after months of stress and strain trying to save the marriage and then realizing that it could not be saved; pushing and cajoling all the way in getting her to actually leave the apartment. It took several years for me to regain enough self-esteem to allow myself to be happy again. In the interim, my ex would call and ask me if I was happy, whatever that meant; all along assuring me that she was "happy, so very happy, the happiest I've ever been; oh, so happy that I never realized how happy I could be ..." She that protests too much, as the saying goes, is not happy at all!

The envious are not happy unless they are making other people envious.

—*Unknown*

So, many of you may have had similar experiences that have placed happiness or being happy in a different kind of perspective for you, one in which much work must be put forth in order to allow personal happiness to blossom from the mayhem of a bad relationship. His Holiness the Dalai Lama has discussed relationships in his book *The Art of Happiness* (Riverhead Books, 1998), and he states that it is important for people who are trying to understand relationship issues to understand the basic underlying nature of the relationship itself.

I think that if one wants to be happy with someone else, a meeting of the minds, so to speak, needs to come out of a mutual understanding of who each person is and what each brings to the table of the other. I am not one to recommend that people fight like cats and dogs and then continuously enjoy the fun of making up afterward. That takes too much out of you, dealing with the stress that results from this type of conflict. Woody Allen has been quoted as stating, "Marriage is the death of hope!" Hope and faith are both parts of any relationship and require work to put them together to make a happy relationship. Many relationships look like a placid flowing river with no ripples on the surface, slowly ambling along glittering happy thoughts in the sunlight; however, underneath there is a torrent of fast-flowing molecules careening off rocks and hitting many obstacles in its efforts to make its way to the sea. If we are to be happy, our relationships have to be solid and stable enough so that careening off the obstacles and vicissitudes of life can slow us down but cannot destroy the integrity of our total substance.

I love the numerous book titles about happiness that are available now, such as *The Joys of Happiness; The Art of Happiness; True Happiness; Stumbling on Happiness; Stairway to Happiness; Happiness Quantified; The Morality of Happiness; The Book of Happiness; Happiness is Always a Delusion;* and, *The Happiness Trap,* to name a few. Looking at these titles, one can see that there is no one definition of happiness or of being happy.

As I previously stated, I think happiness and being happy is an intangible state of being that we each have to be called upon to define for ourselves. To think that someone would question the morality of being happy or the fact that the state of happiness is a delusion, making schizophrenics of us all in a sense, is ludicrous. I am willing to qualify, not quantify happiness into different levels of being happy, and that is as far as I will go. The more endorphins we have flowing in our bloodstream, the happier we will feel. Remember the travel slogan, "Don't worry, be happy, and come to Jamaica"? You might assume then if you don't worry about anything then you can be happy. We all have many concerns in life, one of which might be the question, "When will it be our time to be happy?" Better yet, "When is the right time to worry?"

Worrying is not good for any of us, as it promotes stress and negative changes to our physiology. I would rather be concerned and know that I can definitely do something about my happiness by keeping a positive attitude. This will also aid in keeping my dignity as well. The two go hand in hand. People who yell and scream at each other day in and day out, fighting about inane things, not only do not help their positive images of each other, but demote each other's self-esteem, happiness together and dignity. Musician Bob Dylan wrote a song about dignity with a last stanza indicating how difficult it is for some of us to find dignity. The lines read like this: "So many roads, so much at stake, So many dead ends, I'm at the edges of the lake, Sometimes I wonder what it's gonna take, to find dignity."

Dignity is a fleeting moniker because, as the dictionary reminds us, it is a mental state of being worthy of honor or respect (The *Oxford American Desk Dictionary and Thesaurus*, Second Edition). If one cannot find respect for one's self in the present light of others, then dignity falls into the dark side of being, thereby becoming an intangible state, one that requires searching the soul deeply in order to find the light again. This definition reminds me of a friend of mine who died in his nineties. He once told me that he had lost his light into the dignity of himself. As he was dying, he felt that he had no more dignity left. He measured this state of dignity by physical means rather than a state of mind. He also and made reference to the fact that he could no longer cook or clean for himself, nor could he help his wife who was suffering from the ravages of Alzheimer's disease. Further, he couldn't even walk without the aid of a cane, walker, or caregiver. "So where is my dignity?" he would ask me.

I told him that he still had his sense of dignity; this intangible state of being happy about what he did have, who he was, and what he had accomplished. He also had his family, who came to see him regularly trying to promote his health and general state of happiness. He told me that this was the trick, the guise, under which he was living then: the idea that he was staying alive, not taking his own life, in the face of keeping others happy. The people he was referring to were those individuals in his family and friends who came to him, as a pilgrimage of sorts, humbling themselves at his feet, singing his praises for his life's work and deeds. To him, it was all a sham and he allowed it to continue in order to make others happy. Inside, he lived in the dark world of only existing with the knowledge of his imminent death and inability to function as he had before, keeping him from regaining his dignity.

I have a neighbor who is about eighty years young. She always greets me with a large smile and happy words. No day goes by when I do see her that she does not ask me, "When will you be on TV again?" (So she can watch me). She thinks I am an actor since she saw me interviewed once many years ago on the local news about new innovations in technology for dentistry. This woman was a nurse and had the misfortune of going over a cliff in her car, falling at least three hundred feet to the sea and surviving. Her brain is not fully functioning, but she holds her sense of dignity well and cares for herself most of the time. She is happy and that may be a function of her brain damage as well as body chemistry, but at times I think that she knows what she is all about and fools everyone with this act of being somewhere else mentally.

The point I am trying to make here is that in spite of my neighbor's physical or mental frailties, she still exhibits respect for herself and others. She still gives a wave and a smile in passing no matter how innocent or how small they may be. These gestures are what they are: an example of sharing goodwill, happiness, and dignity with someone else, plain and simple just like my neighbor. If an eighty-year-old mentally and physically challenged person can do this, so can you. I challenge you to this task.

> *People are like stained-glass windows. They sparkle and shine when the sun is out, but when the darkness sets in, their true beauty is revealed only if there is a light from within.*
>
> —Dr. Elisabeth Kübler-Ross, Psychiatrist

What I have learned from older people who never acted their age about happiness and dignity is that in order to have these experiences, one must be able to convey them to others. Couple this with love, respect for self and others, as well as self-love and wisdom, and anyone can find happiness and dignity in their lives if they look for it.

Recently, I met an eighty-one-years-young woman who spent her entire life taking care of her husband and his business. He has passed on now and he was a fine artist for over fifty years. I asked her what she learned from being his wife and from his work. She first told me that she did not think that she was old. She emphatically stated that "getting old was for sissies!" she told me the majority of her friends were younger people.

She reads constantly, she gardens and takes pride in her garden and the beauty she has created around her. She takes trips and she studies life, both the present and the past in order to understand herself. She is alone and happy about it. We are always alone from birth until death, at least inside our own heads, with our own thoughts and our own visions of today and tomorrow. Happiness for her is ever present, in spite of the physical ills that she fights to overcome. Dignity remains a solid feature of her life because she has not allowed herself to go without it. Having been through World War II, where she may have felt little to no happiness or dignity, this woman now finds pride in both her deceased husband's work and her own work and life.

I am finding many examples of similar instances in the number of elderly people I have counseled who have gone through years of sadness, personal loss, the horrors of war, physical and mental hardships, poverty and abuse and are now exploring ways, in their final years of life, to find happiness and take pride in what they have accomplished. It comes faster for some than others because some of us may have a better handle on what it is we want from life. I have always been an advocate of making my own opportunities, but this takes much thought, planning, visioning and work. Without these attributes it may be difficult to find what you are looking for because things don't just generally happen unless you were born with a sliver spoon in your mouth. Mine was plastic!

> *Seven gifts my mother gave me: 1. The gift of right: if mamma saw a wrong she righted it. 2. The gift of friendliness: making people happier than they were before 3. The gift of rose-colored vision: mamma liked for the flowers, not the weeds. 4. The gift of fun: mamma gave us the best gift a mother can—her time. 5. The gift of understanding: she was always trying to solve people's problems or at least listen to them. 6. The gift of thoughtfulness: she didn't wait for something special, she just did kind acts any time she saw the need. 7. The gift of respect: when you help to inch your fellow man along on that struggle to dignity, he*

loves you for it. Seven gifts? I could list seven hundred gifts my mother gave me. Gifts not boxed and ribboned. Not always noticed or even appreciated at the time. But a part of us. Forever.

—*Meredith Willson, American composer*

Chapter 11

The End Is Only the Beginning and Then Some

Rome was not built in a day and either was the concept of Man; that is, the ability of Man to rise above other animals to think, reason, cry, grow older, and prosper. One can find many aspects of the aging process that may impede its progress, change its course, embellish its function, or carry it along in good stead. Making peace with the aging process involves a lot of work, understanding, knowledge about being human and all the frailties that go along with the so-called ultimate human challenge: acceptance. Making friends with the aging process involves a consensus and acknowledgment of getting older and making compromises as you age.

I don't think there is a way to overlook getting older. The physical signs and symptoms are too prevalent and are constant reminders that all things change, including you and me and everyone we know, unless we die at an early age. Even the dying process brings on changes and challenges we need to try to accept for ultimate peace of mind. So, coming to grips with getting older is what is necessary for making peace with the process and ultimate acceptance of who we are and what is going to become of us.

All too often I have heard from peers, "I am old." I don't see them as old. I see them as aging. I tell all of them that being or getting old is a state of mind, and aging is a state of being, based on awareness. If you go about labeling yourself as old, thinking that you are old; then you *will be* old! It helps to be positive during this process and in turn, this helps gain acceptance from your mind and psyche about aging; in essence getting older gracefully.

You can't help getting older, but you don't have to get old.
—George Burns, American comedian

Many people approach what I call the "boomer triangle," that is, adjusting to each stage of the aging ladder—fifty to sixty-five and then to eighty-five—finding these times in the aging process difficult to adjust to, stressful, and challenging to both their physical abilities and emotional capabilities. Many people may be hindered by the presence of systemic or chronic disease, while others may be obsessed with thoughts about changing their appearance with plastic surgery or becoming reclusive. Botox use is rampant among the boomer generation. It is amazing to me that so many people would allow this toxin to be injected into their faces on a regular basis just to keep the wrinkles down! If you have seen someone on Botox then you would have noticed the lack of smile lines and expressions with a blank stare or a placid wax-like look, because the toxin keeps the muscles from working to some degree, preventing the flexing of the skin to form wrinkles. This is not what I was alluding to when I titled this book *A New Wrinkle*.

My objective in writing this book was to liberate people's minds about the aging process, tempering the metamorphosis of getting older so that people would be more at ease knowing some of the things to look for along the way, and bringing hope to those who wish to remain healthy, wealthy, and wise throughout their lifespan. Who could ask for anything better than a primer on aging? I must admit—since so many people have asked me "What do you know about the aging process at your age?"—that I feel honored to have been able to write this book with the limited, perceived knowledge and information people seem to think that I have. I feel that I have been entrusted with these stories and personal experiences by the many elders whom I have been privileged enough to come to know for over sixty years, each of whom has had a relationship with me in some manner or another.

I have gleaned information and knowledge from these wonderful people of all makes and models, at different levels of aging and at varying stages of life, so that I could write my book using the wisdom I have accumulated as a reference tool for others. In doing so, I keep the memory of all those people I have known and cherished alive. Don't be fooled by the thinking that there may not be wisdom in all people. You just have to look and listen for it to arise. I think I have done that deed. However, some people wouldn't recognize a wise man if he was wearing a sign that said, "I'm a wise man!" People's perception about others is what he or she will believe in the long run, and no one will be able to change this thinking unless people allow themselves to be educated. This is all part of the acceptance stage of getting older. None of us will change our perceptions about aging unless we are able to understand some of the ramifications that create this place in our lives. In order to make peace within ourselves, we must learn to be at peace with the changes that confront us as time goes by.

Letting go of all preconceived notions about getting older would be a good first step. Just let the processes happen but don't neglect taking care of yourself. Giving in to the aging process will help you with the acceptance part of getting older. However, some of us never grow up.

Stifling the inner child in you due to getting older is a no-no. All of us need that inner child to keep perspective about where we came from, maintaining our sense of wonder and creativity, our ability to have fun, and to be able to play as well as to keep us young minded. These things we need to carry with us wherever we go, calling upon them to help us as we age. We need to be able to laugh at ourselves and not take life so seriously, even in the face of crisis and tragedy. We need to learn to move on through the vicissitudes of life, getting over ourselves in the process. Being stuck in the mud, so to speak, is some place I do not want to be. I use this term of speech to indicate not being able to change with respect to the rigors of the aging process. Also, not being able to call upon your inner strengths, which would include your inner child, would keep you from growing wiser; but not necessarily keep you from growing older.

> *Wisdom: To live in the present, plan for the future, profit from the past.*
>
> —*Unknown*

Knowing Who We Are

Much of what has been covered in this book is material to educate you about how to be prepared for changes in your life around getting older. I wanted you to be especially aware of things that you might not expect to have happen to you when you either grow up, in the literal sense, or reach the end of the line within the realm of your individual family's forcing you to deal with specific issues around the aging process. This book will hopefully help you cope and compromise with others who have had negative experiences in their own lives, or who may be negative influences on your positive aging process.

I think that through all of our sets of experiences at some point in time we must sit down and think about who we are, where we came from, and where we are going in a logical manner. This will place things in perspective for us as we age. Knowing these things will allow us to chart a course for the future because we now have reached a point in time that enables us to be selective about ourselves; having learned who we will become and what we want to achieve. People with families will want to evaluate how they fit into the family and where the family should be in due course. If something happens in the family, then we will know how to help with the challenge by being prepared. The colloquial phrase, "Know thyself and to thine own self be true," helps us to gauge how we are able to act and react to situations that test us in our journey of aging.

We all must learn to love ourselves. This is one of the greatest gifts we can give to ourselves; again, only learning to give this gift away in the end. In giving love away, we find a higher meaning in our own lives. Having faith, spiritual values, and something of a higher power to believe in will give each of us an added boost in coping with life and with aging. Each of us is charged with the responsibility of helping ourselves and helping others as well. That is why we each, hopefully, have two hands: one for helping ourselves and one for helping others.

It goes without saying, that growing older is difficult. Some of us never really wanted to take responsibility for ourselves, and yet we were forced to do so in the process of growing up. Many people were forced to grow up at an early age and missed out on the nurturing they required to fulfill the hierarchy of needs necessary to develop a good sense of self-connectedness to being loved, with reference to Abraham Maslow's theories of a greater hierarchy of needs. His theory, developed in 1943, suggests that certain levels of needs want to be satisfied, one before the other, before complete actualization of the self occurs. The levels are: physiological needs such as breathing, food, water, sex, sleep, homeostasis and excretion; safety needs such as security of body, employment, resources, morality, family, health, and property; love and belonging needs such as friendship, family, and sexual intimacy; esteem needs such as self-esteem, confidence, achievement, respect for others, and respect by others; and finally, self-actualization needs such as morality, creativity, spontaneity, problem solving, lack of prejudice and acceptance of facts.

Not having this nurturing process, many individuals have found it even more difficult to survive in the real world because they do not know what love is with respect to the greater hierarchy, having received very little of it while in their childhood years. This situation makes it difficult for these individuals to relate to others in later life, adding to stress levels as well as physical and mental disease states.

Loving yourself, then, is imperative in helping you get through each day. I tell my clients to look into the mirror each day and repeat the following mantra, "No one can hurt me because I love myself too much." I learned this from my friend Vera, who has had many hardships in her own life to cope with and overcome. I guess being your own champion helps bolster the hurt ego, until we can find an accomplice, of sorts, who will compliment our being as a soul mate or companion in our journey; even if it is ourselves, metaphysically speaking. Learning to receive love, not just provide it, is a basic statement about acceptance of one's self.

A Short Story

I had a client not long ago in his eighties who was beginning the long, arduous journey of living with dementia. His family, mainly his daughter, was concerned about him, having just discovered that his entire life had been a lie—a lie about who he was and what he had accomplished. The family was hurt, angry, riddled with guilt, and ashamed after finding out their father had lied about his entire life, including his military service achievements. The father, plagued by loss of memories, could not understand that he did anything wrong because the memory that he did have, the one that was false, had become his reality. This was all the old man had. This was his past, present and future all rolled into one.

This man was probably a victim of early separation from his mother and family. Having missed out on the nurturing that he needed to enable him to become whole, Charlie (a pseudonym) was emotionally lost. Living his lie was what he had learned to do in order to make himself more important in the eyes of those who knew him, especially his family. His actions were an effort to gain love and respect for who he was, even though Charlie had no idea who he was at this point in his life. Deep down inside, Charlie was an insecure little boy, lost in the mire of a sinking life with only the circumnavigation of the truth to keep him whole.

I stressed to his daughter that he was unable to change and that things were only going to get worse regarding the dementia. Charlie was still driving and he would go out daily to a local restaurant, find people to talk to, tell his story, buy them all meals and rounds, making himself the center of attention. This is just what Charlie needed to fill the emptiness of an unknown self inside his unconscious mind. At one point, Charlie's daughter had to take away his credit cards and place him on an allowance. I recommended that they consider taking away his driver's license as well as getting him a caregiver. I never knew what happened to Charlie in the end, but I do know that he was happy and loved the life he made up for himself more than anything he had, other than his dog.

Perception is people's reality no matter who they are or what it is they think about. Unless people are educated about life and the inevitable future, people's reality will not change. If we let our desires guide us into our future without understanding what we need to do to prepare for it, then no matter what happens we are slaves to our perceptions. This may be all right for some of us who might be experiencing cognitive decline, but for the majority it is important to get a handle on life, and how one can enjoy the fruits of one's labors with respect to aging. No one is immune from disease, taxes, costs of living, basic needs, or death. No one gets out of this world alive! We may be given several chances to get it right, but basically we only have one time around as ourselves. In this case, why not make your life exciting, useful, fun, loving, spiritual, full of laughter, healthy, worthwhile, productive, and beneficial to all concerned?

He, who has the last laugh, lasts.

—Unknown

I have known many people who have financial wealth, but do not experience emotional happiness. Some of these people have all the luxuries in the world and more. These people are in their sixties, seventies, and eighties and are basically healthy, but suffer from the insecurity of not having enough love or friends in their lives. Without people to share life with, we cannot validate our own self-worth. When I asked my ninety-year-young friend about finding the meaning of life before he passed away, he turned to me and said, "If you want to find out the meaning of your life, ask someone else!" a most profound comment and one that still reverberates in my brain daily. I think that he was attempting to point out that we should let other people judge us as to whether we have made a difference to them. If we don't know, then we need to ask. I think he was right for the most part, but I also think that each of us knows whether we have made a difference to someone else. Empirically speaking, I think that my friend was looking at the broader picture of the meaning of one's life.

President Jimmy Carter stated in his book *The Virtues of Aging* (Ballantine Books, 1998), that in our later years we should all come to realize that "the simple things that comprise success include our own happiness, satisfaction, peace, joy, and a sense of being worthy." We all need to have people we trust, admire, love, and respect that we can ask to be our mirrors regarding our accomplishments. Everyone needs positive feedback to feel good, but we also should demand criticism enough to allow us to process where we need to improve. What can each of us do to make our lives meaningful as we age? Is it enough just to do good deeds? I think we all need our story tellers, the people we surround ourselves with who can tell our legacies: the deeds and messages we leave behind so others can remember us.

Epilogue

I have spent many years in school learning to be a better person and a more educated individual so that I could impart what I have learned to benefit others. I am, as you are reading this book, the sum total of all my experiences.

What does that mean in effect? It means that who you are as a person is the identity you get from your history, the relationships you have had with others in your past, present and future, the education you have experienced, the accumulation and subsequent understanding you have of your emotional and physical needs, including but not limited to pain, suffering, joy, good times, bad times, epiphanies, moments that take your breath away, memories, friends, family, enemies, angels, a higher belief and the changes you have learned to accept or bring to a compromise.

Each of these entities allows you the ability to synthesize something useful in your life due to the potpourri of ingredients that make you who you are. Most of us reach older age and want to place much of this legacy behind us, waiting for the inevitable to occur; not realizing that what we have been through and accomplished is a gift of knowledge and experience for others, waiting to be imparted. These things are a way for us to find ultimate happiness in the world—a true understanding of self and our environment with respect to others. Aging is a process that starts with birth. The only time this process ends is when we die.

Somewhere in the middle we might have an epiphany that we are aging and it is then that we start to get edgy about our mortality. If you have seen the movie *The Bucket List*, you will relate to my statement. Imminent death brings on the overriding desire to do all the things that one might have pushed aside, or put on hold for a while until such time that it was feasible to do them. The slogan, "Time waits for no man," seems to ring a bell here about the expediency of continuing to enhance one's life by learning, doing, teaching, sharing, and not wasting that precious time in the process of aging, no matter where you are in the process. Life is too short to waste on trivialities and not long enough to do all that one wishes they would accomplish in the time they have left on Earth, which is unknown.

We all need our so-called mirrors to help us see what it is we have become and then we need to learn to process this information in order to create a kind of *paint* that we can coat on every one we meet; in essence, allowing others to take away something useful for themselves from us, embellishing their lives in some way as a reflection of our thoughts, our love, and our ideas about growing older in a healthy, useful way.

Our lives then, are moveable canvasses over which we *paint* our ever-changing stories for admiration and display. Our interpretation of what we are and have become stop when the painting is finished; but the interpretation of what we have left behind is now up to the many spectators who are left to figure out what it is we have given them through the art we call our lifetimes. The trick is in slowing down and to know when to stop painting.

> *And the wind said: "May you be as strong as the oak, yet flexible as the birch; may you stand tall as the Redwood,*

live gracefully as the willow; and may you always bear fruit all your days on this earth."

—*Native American prayer*

Laugh a lot, share love a lot, live a lot, get to a place where you know yourself and enjoy life as you know it; let your inner child out to play as well as teach others by sharing your gifts. Above all, have no regrets about how you have lived …

Eric Zane Shapira

Glossary of Terms

A

Acupuncture. An ancient Chinese traditional medical technique utilizing fine needles placed into meridians, or lines running through the body, in order to treat ailments and disease

ADD. Attention Deficit Disorder

ADL. Activities of Daily Living, e.g., brushing one's teeth, dressing, or washing

Adult Day Health Center. A facility that allows respite for caretakers of medically and emotionally disabled adults, whereby the clients can spend most of their day there while their children work

Agape. A deep form of love (from the Greek)

Aging. Showing signs of advancing age; a process

Agnosia. Visual recognition problems

AIDS. Acquired Immune Deficiency Syndrome; a deadly life-threatening viral disease

Alzheimer's disease. A form of dementia and cognitive decline distinguished by the buildup of protein plaque in the brain, loss of inhibitions, and severe, progressive memory loss

Anesthesia. A method for putting a person into an unconscious or unfeeling state of numbness, usually for a surgical or operative procedure of some sort

Aphasia. Difficulty with or lack of speech

Apraxia. Difficulty manually doing things, e.g., buttoning a shirt

A priori. Working from something that is already known or self evident

Archeologist. A scientist of ancient cultures

Arthritis. A disease causing pain and swelling to the joints

Ashkenazi. A specific sect of the Jewish religion with a Mediterranean or Spanish influence

Assisted living. A facility that aids in the life of those who need assisting

Attachment Disorder. A psychological condition predicated upon the loss of parental attachment from childhood, which creates a neurotic need for coupling

Attitude. A way of thinking

Auriculotherapy. A form of acupuncture applied to the outer ear

Autoimmune disease. A disease or illness that is brought on by a phenomenon whereby body tissues are attacked by its own immune system

B

Baby boomer. A person born post World War II between the years of 1946 and 1964

Bandwagon. Extremely popular movement or cause

Benchmark. A standard or reference point

Bonded. A state of being attached, connected mentally, or duty bound to another

Breadwinner. A person within a family who earns a living monetarily

Bubbie. A name for a Jewish grandmother

Bushman. An aboriginal native of southern Africa

C

Cancer. A life-threatening disease caused by a malignant growth tumor of abnormal body cells

Cardiovascular. Pertaining to the heart and associated blood vessels

Caregiver. A person who has the responsibility of taking care of another

Cephalopodan. Having a distinctly tentacled head (literally meaning *head-foot* from the Latin)

Centenarian. A person who has reached 100 years of age

Cerebral cortex. The outer portion of the brain consisting of gray matter

Change. A constant process of moderation or alteration resulting in becoming different

Chi. A word of Chinese origin that means the interplay of two forces that make up the material governing the universe; balance between essential harmony and health of the individual

Chiropractic. Manipulative treatment of mechanical disorders of the joints, especially of the spinal column

Cholinesterase. An enzyme found in the body, primarily at nerve endings, that catalyzes the hydrolysis (splitting) of acetylcholine into acetic acid and chlorine; this stops the stimulation of muscles fibers

Chronic disease. A pathological condition that persists or lasts for a long time

Chrysalis. A cocoon, or wrap, supporting the makings of a butterfly

Cognition. The state of being aware or having knowledge

Colonoscopy. A medical test designed to view the inside of the colon with a scope and camera

COPD. Chronic obstructive pulmonary disease

Corporate. Forming one body of many individuals

Cortisol. A chemical hormone manufactured within the body at the onset of stress that stimulates increased blood sugar, increased blood pressure, and the autonomic nervous system

Coumadin. A drug, such as heparin, that thins the blood

CPR. Cardiopulmonary resuscitation; an emergency procedure to bring a person back to life from heart failure or respiratory arrest

Creativity. An imaginative process that spawns new ideas about things; resourceful and inventive

CT scan; Computerized tomography. A clinical test that allows for the vision of body parts by a radiographic sectioning of the x-ray film through the body part being examined

CVA. Cerebral vascular accident; a stroke

D

Dalai Lama. The revered, exiled religious leader of Tibet known for his wisdom and preaching's

Dehydration. Reduction of water content

Delusion. A false belief or impression that may be a symptom of a psychological disorder

Dementia. A type of disease related to memory loss and senility from a variety of causes

Depression. A state of extreme melancholy, often with clinical or physical symptoms such as crying and isolation

Diabetes. A systemic endocrine disease of the pancreas that affects the ability of cells to digest sugars due to decreased insulin production in the pancreas or the inability of cells to absorb insulin

Digestive tract. That part of the body where food is converted into material suitable for assimilation for synthesis of tissues and liberation of energy, e.g., stomach, small intestine, large intestine

Dignity. A state of self-respect and high regard

Dios de las Muertes, Los. The Days of the Dead; a Latin holiday celebrated around Halloween, which commemorates those that have died in celebration of life

Disability. Physical or mental incapacity

Don Quixote. A literary mythical person who was known for fighting windmills, which he perceived as giants, in Spain

Drug interaction. The pharmacological result, either desirable or undesirable, of drugs interacting with themselves or other drugs, with endogenous physiologic chemical agents, with components of the diet, and with chemicals used in diagnostic tests or the results of such tests

Durable power of healthcare. A legal document that specifies how one would like to be treated should it become necessary for someone else to make medical and ethical decisions for them due to a medical condition that renders them incapable of doing so

E

Economist. A person who studies the wealth and resources of a community

E-health. The body of health information found on the Internet

Elder. A person who is over the age of eighty-five years; connotes wisdom

Empathic. A state of showing empathy or a nonjudgmental paraphrasing of what someone is saying

Endocrine. One of the systems of the body responsible for producing specific hormones, which are secreted directly into the blood stream

Endorphin. A chemical made of opioid peptides originally isolated in the brain but since found in many parts of the body, which cause physiologic reactions that can produce feelings of euphoria and excitement

Epinephrine. A catecholamine that is the chief neurohormone of the adrenal medulla of most species; causes many physiologic reactions in both stress and normal function; used for anaphylactic shock and allergic disorders as an injection

Epiphany. A moment of profound insight

Erectile dysfunction. The inability to have or sustain an erection of the penis or male sex organ

Executive dysfunction. The inability to think properly or take action when it comes to things like driving a car, working, and making clear decisions

F

Family map. A genogram of sorts, showing the traits, habits, and addictions of family members as well as the patterns of birth and death cycles

Fear. An emotional state causing heightened anxiety with possibly no identifiable stimulus

Foreplay. Stimulative sexual activity preceding sexual intercourse

Fountain of Youth. A mythical place that supposedly harbored the waters of long life; the place that Ponce de Leon, Spanish explorer, spent most of his life looking for in obscurity

Free radical. A radical in its uncombined state; an atom or atom group carrying an unpaired electron and no charge. These may be short-lived, highly active intermediates in various reactions in living tissue, notable in photosynthesis; but it is theorized that these also act in human tissues to promote heart disease, cancer, Alzheimer's disease, Parkinson's disease, and rheumatoid arthritis. They may be introduced to the body through eating impure foods, smoking or inhaling environmental pollutants or exposure to UV radiation, and also occur naturally within the body as a result of a metabolic process.

G

Gene. A functional unit of heredity that occupies a specific place on a chromosome, is capable of reproducing itself exactly at each cell division, and directs the formation of an enzyme or other protein. 20,000-25,000 genes in human DNA

Geriatrician. A physician who specializes in the field of aging and its disease states

Gerontologist. One who specializes in gerontology, or the study of aging, its processes and diseases

Gerontology. The scientific study of the process and problems of aging

GPS. Global positioning system; a mechanism that tells location by longitude and latitude at any given point of time using satellite technology

Grass roots. A fundamental level or source; usually from the bottom up

Grief. A normal emotional response to an external loss; distinguished from a depressive disorder since it usually subsides after a reasonable time

Guided imagery. A technique similar to hypnosis, which guides a client through suggested images or visualizations that may be helpful in ridding the client of negative influence, post traumatic stress, anxiety, and various bad habits

Guru. A Hindu spiritual leader or head of a religious sect; basically an influential teacher

H

Happyness. (purposeful misspelling) A state of being happy or showing pleasure, delight, enjoyment, joy, gladness, high spirits

Hippocampus. That portion of the brain that is thought to harbor new information and memories

HIV. Human Immunodeficiency Virus

Home Health Agency. Any number of organizations that support the use of trained employees used to take care of aging individuals who may be physically or mentally challenged in some way

Homeostasis. The state of equilibrium (balance between opposing pressures) in the body with respect to various functions and to the chemical compositions of the fluids and tissues; the process through which bodily equilibrium is maintained

Hormone. A chemical substance, formed in one organ or part of the body and carried in the blood to another organ or part, which can alter the functional activity, and sometimes structure, of just one organ or of various numbers of them

Hospice. A worldwide movement founded in England by a physician, Dame Cecily Saunders, which supports the care of the dying and their families on all levels

Humanitarian. A person who seeks to promote human welfare

Hypnosis. An artificially induced trancelike state, resembling somnambulism (sleep walking) and having scientific validity, in which the subject is highly susceptible to suggestion, oblivious to all else, and responds readily to the commands of the hypnotist. A process tapping the unconscious mind

Hypertrophy. General increase in bulk of a part or organ, not due to tumor formation

Hypothalamus. The underside and middle region of the diencephalon forming the walls of the underside half of the third ventricle (a portion within the center of the brain); thought to function as a primary center for the function of the autonomic nervous system as well as playing a role in neural mechanisms underlying moods and motivational states

I

ICU. Intensive care unit of a hospital; where acute postsurgical or endangered individuals are taken for care

Independent contractor. A person who works for themselves under the supervision of another; not an employee per se

Infarct. An area of necrosis (dead tissue) resulting from a sudden insufficiency of arterial or venous blood supply

Immortal. Living forever or famous for all time

Immune system. The specific system or a specific part of the human body that fights or protects against infection; normally given over to the white blood cells and other antibody containing factors in the blood serum

Impairment. A physical or mental defect at the level of a body system or organ

Infection. Multiplication of parasitic organisms (bacteria, virus, or other foreign animals or protein bodies that cause disease) within the body

Intimacy. The state of making oneself known to another at the deepest levels; possibly sexual

J

Journey. An expedition; the act of going from one place to another (this can be physical or mental)

L

Legacy. Things handed down by a predecessor

Leukemia. Progressive proliferation of abnormal white blood cells in the blood in increased amounts which can cause death

Loch Ness. A lake in northern Scotland believed to harbor the mythical Loch Ness monster

Longevity. Long life

M

Mariposa. Butterfly (Spanish)

Maslow's hierarchy of needs. A theory in psychology depicted as a pyramid of five levels associated with various learned or innate entities that, if completed, create a sense of self-esteem; theorized by Abraham Maslow

Medicare/Medicaid. A federal mandate that allows for those individuals over the age of sixty-five years to partake of financial benefits for healthcare and sustenance assistance; Medicaid is found on the state level and allows for financial benefits for younger people and families as well

Meditation. A method of relaxation, deep thought, and contemplation

Melanoma. A form of deadly skin cancer

Memory. The mental faculty by which things are recalled; remembrance of stored thoughts and information in the brain

Mental health. A scientific field that encompasses the treatment of psychological disorders and anxiety; also indicates a state of mind

Meridian. A corresponding line or lines that divide the body into regions depicting a map for the use of acupuncture points that are the focus of needles used to cure specific diseases or conditions of the body

Methyl trexate. A drug to treat rheumatoid arthritis and certain forms of leukemia; anti-inflammatory medication

Micromanage. A term used to denote the fastidious way a manger manages a business or employees by being involved in everything that goes on to the point of being excessive

Migraine. A symptom complex occurring periodically and characterized by pain in the head (usually unilateral), vertigo, nausea and vomiting, photophobia (sensitivity to light), and scintillating appearances of light

Mild cognitive impairment. A beginning state of memory loss and dementia characterized by acknowledgement of being forgetful about things on a constant basis

MMPI. Minnesota Multi-Phasic Inventory; a psychological test that indicates personality traits

Morphine. An opioid derivative used as a strong pain medication, sedative, and anxiolytic (anti-anxiety medication); can be highly addicting

MRI. An abbreviation for Magnetic Resonance Imaging; a form of radiographic analysis

Multiple myeloma. An uncommon disease that occurs more frequently in men than in women and is associated with anemia, hemorrhage, recurrent infections, and weakness; regarded as a malignant neoplasm that originates in bone marrow and involves chiefly the skeleton

N

Nani. A Yiddish word referring to a grandmother

Neurologist. A physician who specializes in the study of the nervous system, diagnosis and treatment of muscular disorders; the central, peripheral, and autonomic nervous systems; the neuromuscular junction; and muscle

NMDA-Receptor Antagonist. An abbreviation for N-methyl D-aspartate, an excitotoxic amino acid used to identify a specific subset of glutamine receptors in the treatment of memory loss

O

Octogenarian. A person who has reached eighty years of age

P

Parkinson's disease. A neurological syndrome usually resulting from deficiency of the neurotransmitter dopamine as the consequence of degenerative, vascular, or inflammatory changes in the basal ganglia of the brain; characterized by rhythmical muscular tremors, rigidity of movement, festination, droopy posture, masklike facies, shaking palsy, and trembling palsy

Pediatrician. A physician who specializes in the study and treatment of children in health and disease during development from birth through adolescence

Peer counselor. A person who counsels others of the same age bracket or ilk

Pestilence. A fatal epidemic disease or plague

Phoenix. A mythical bird, the only one of its kind, that burned itself on a funeral pyre and rose from the ashes to live again through another cycle

Physician. A medical doctor or healer

Physiology. The science of the functions of living organisms and their parts

Pituitary. The master endocrine gland of the body whose hormones are responsible for growth, sexual function, childbirth, and lactation, among other functions

Peritoneal cavity. The serous sac, consisting of mesothelium and a thin layer of irregular connective tissue, that lines the abdominal cavity and covers most of the viscera (organs) contained therein

PMS. An abbreviation for premenstrual syndrome; characterized by irregular menstrual periods due to hormonal changes at mid-life and extreme mood changes and hot flashes

Power of attorney. A document that allows one person to have the power and control over legal, financial, and business matters of another

Prehistoric. Of or relating to a time before written records; a time of dinosaurs and cave men and cave women

Protocol. Official formality and etiquette; rules or standards of behavior, conventions, customs and form

Protoplasm. Living matter, the substance of which animal and vegetable cells are formed; the total cell material

Psyche. Term for the subjective aspects of the mind, self, soul; the psychological or spiritual as distinct from the bodily nature of persons

Psychiatrist. A physician who diagnoses and treats people with mental disorders

Psychologist. A specialist in psychology; the scholarly discipline and science concerned with the behavior of humans and animals and related mental and physiological processes

Psychoses. A mental and behavioral disorder causing gross distortion or disorganization of a person's mental capacity, affective response, and capacity to recognize reality, communicate, and relate to others to the degree of interfering with the person's capacity to cope with the ordinary demands of everyday life

Q

Quality. A degree of excellence

Quantity. Property of things that is measured

R

RA. An abbreviation for rheumatoid arthritis; a systemic disease occurring more often in women, which affects connective tissue with dominant clinical manifestations involving many joints, especially of the hands and feet, leading to deformities and disability

RN. An abbreviation for registered nurse

S

Schizophrenia. A new term used to describe the "original" disease label of dementia praecox; a psychosis, characterized by a disorder in perception, content of thought, and thought processes (hallucinations and delusions), and extensive withdrawal of the individual's interest from other people and the outside world, and the investment of it in his own

Sciatica. Pain in the lower back and hip radiating down the back of the thigh into the leg, initially attributed to sciatic nerve dysfunction, but now known to usually be due to herniated lumbar disk compromising L5 or S1 roots; continuous disease, sciatic neuralgia

Selenium. A metallic element chemically similar to sulfur, which is toxic in large quantities; required for glutathione peroxidase and a few other enzymes to function properly; helps in the preservation of cells and longevity

Senility. A general term for a variety of mental disorders occurring in old age which consist of two broad categories, organic and psychological disorders

Shivah. A ceremony in the Hebrew faith that revolves around the death of a Jewish person; observed for one week and requires at least thirteen Jewish men to complete

Statistics. The science of collecting and analyzing numerical data; any systematic collection or presentation of such facts

Steroids. A large family of chemical substances usually manufactured in the adrenal glands, comprising many hormones, body constituents, and drugs; can increase muscle mass, reduce inflammation, and allergic reactions

STD. An acronym for sexually transmitted diseases

Surgeon General. A physician appointed by the president of the United States to oversee the health aspects of the general population within the United States

SWOT. An acronym for: strengths, weaknesses, opportunities, and threats; used in business or any profession where one needs to form a strategic or business plan

Syphilis. An acute and chronic infectious disease cased by Treponema pallidum and transmitted by direct contact, usually through sexual intercourse

Systemic. Relating to a system; specifically somatic, relating to the entire organism as distinguished from any of its individual parts

T

TB. An abbreviation for tuberculosis; a specific disease caused by the presence of Mycobacterium tuberculosis, which may affect almost any tissue or organ of the body, the most common seat of the disease being the lungs

Thalamus. The large, ovoid mass of gray matter that forms the larger dorsal subdivision of the diencephalon of the brain, which functions to retain and process new memories

Theory of Relativity. Developed by Albert Einstein; relates energy to the mass of a particle or atom, times the speed of light in centimeters squared: $E=mc^2$

Thomas Edison. A famous American inventor known for inventing the electric light, among other things

TIA. Acronym for transient ischemic attack (or mini-stroke)

Transition. Passing or change from one place, state, condition, style to another

Triglycerides. A fatty acid made up of mono- and diglycerides; found in the body and can form plaque on arterial walls

Trust. A legal document that describes how one's personal property, and money will pass to ones descendents once death occurs; confidence, reliance, firm belief in the reliability, truth, or strength of a person or thing

U

USO. United Service Organization; an American non-profit organization that supports military personnel and their families throughout the world

V

Validate. To acknowledge or confirm that something is acceptable

Viagra. A drug used to help with erectile dysfunction with the ability to cause an erection due to its effects on the dilation of blood vessels in the penis

Vitamin. One of a group of organic substances, present in minute amounts in natural foodstuffs, which are essential to normal metabolism; insufficient amounts in the diet may cause deficiency diseases

W

Will. A legal document that specifies how one's property will be distributed after death and to whom

Wisdom. Experience and knowledge together with the power of applying them; state of being wise

Wrinkle. A line of experience or mark of due diligence; a slight crease in the skin produced by age or creases in clothing caused by bunching

X

Y

Yiddish. A language created with a mixture of German and Slavic languages; used by the Jewish people during World War II so as not to be understood by the Nazis

Yin-yang. In ancient Chinese thought, the concept of two complimentary and opposing influences, yin and yang, underlying and controlling all nature, the aim of Chinese medicine being to produce proper balance between them

Z

Zymurgy. A branch of applied chemistry related to fermentation

Zymurgy's First Law of Inertial Dynamics. Once you open a can of worms, you will need a larger can to put them back into

Related Reading

Albom, Mitch *Tuesdays with Morrie*. NY: Doubleday Publishing, 1997

Bortz II, MD, Walter, M. *Dare To Be 100*. Fireside Publishing, 1996

Bortz II, MD, Walter, M. *Living Longer for Dummies*. Hungry Minds, Inc Publishing,   2001

Bridges, William *Transitions*. Perseus Books, 1980

Callanan,RN, Maggie, and Kelley, Patrice *Final Gifts, Understanding the Special   Awareness, Needs, and Communications of the Dying*. Bantam Books, 1997

Carter, Jimmy *The Virtues of Aging*. The Ballantine Publishing Group, 1998

Casarjian, Robin *Forgiveness: A Bold Choice for a Peaceful Heart*. Bantam Books, 1992

Chopra, MD, Deepak *Ageless Body, Timeless Mind*. Harmony Books, 1993

Corey, Marianne Schneider and Corey, Gerald *Becoming a Helper*. Brooks/Cole Publishing, 2003

Cousins, Norman *Anatomy of an Illness*. Bantam Books, 1979

Crain, William *Theories of Development, Concepts and Applications.* Prentice Hall Publishing, 2000

DeSpelder, Lynne Ann & Strickland, Albert Lee *The Last Dance, Encountering Death and Dying.* Mayfield Publishing Company, 1999

Dollenmore, Doug *The Doctors Book of Home Remedies for Seniors.* Prevention Books, Rodale Press, 1999

Doraiswamy, M.D., P. Murali, & Gwyther, M.S.W., Lisa P., *The Alzheimer's Action Plan. NY: St. Martin's Press,* 2008

Dychtwald, PhD, Ken and Flower, Joe *Age Wave.* Bantam Books, 1990

Ellis, Neenah *If I Live To Be 100, Lessons from the Centenarians.* Crown Publishers, 2002

Erikson, Erik H. *Identity and the Life Cycle.* W.W. Norton Publishing, 1980

Feil, MSW, ACSW, Naomi *The Validation Breakthrough, Simple Techniques for Communicating with People with "Alzheimer's-Type Dementia.* Health Professions Press, 1993

Frankl, Viktor, E. *Man's Search for Meaning.* Simon and Schuster Publishers, 1962

Gates, Bill *The Road Ahead.* New York: Viking Penguin Publishers, 1995-96

Gibran, Kahlil *A Tear and A Smile*, translated by H.N. Nahmud. NY: Alfred A. Knopf Publisher, 1992

Hayflick, PhD, Leonard *How and Why We Age.* Ballantine Books, 1996

Hanh, Thich Nhat, *Breathe, You Are Alive: Sutra on the Full Awareness of Breathing.* Parallax Press, 1996

Hendin, David *Death as a Fact of Life*. W.W. Norton & Company, 1984

Lama, Dahli, His Holiness and Cutler, Howard, M.D. *The Art of Happiness*. Riverhead Books, 1998

Luskin, Fred, Dr. *Forgive for Good*. San Francisco: Harper Publishers, Inc., 2002

MacDonald, Shari Humor for the Heart. Howard Publishing, 2000

May, Rollo, *Meaning of Anxiety. Norton, W.W. & Company, Inc., 1996*

McKay, PhD, Matthew, Davis, PhD, Martha & Fanning, Patrick *How To Communicate*. MJF Books, 1983

Neruda, Pablo *The Yellow Heart*, translated by Wm O'Daly. Washington: Copper Canyon Press, 1990

Paige, Leroy "Satchel," *Maybe I'll Pitch Forever*. University of Nebraska Press, 1986

Petras, Kathryn and Ross *Age Doesn't Matter Unless You're a Cheese*. Workman Publishing, 2002

Remen, MD, Rachel Naomi *My Grandfather's Blessings*. Riverhead Books, 2000

Rosenfeld, MD, Isadore *Live Now Age Later*. Warren Books, 1999

Rosetree, Rose *Wrinkles Are God's Makeup*. Women's Intuition Worldwide, LLC, Publishing, 2003

Siegel, MD, Bernie *Love, Medicine and Miracles*. NY: Harper & Row Publishers, Inc., 1986

Shacter-Shalomi, Zalman and Miller, Ronald *From Aging to Saging*. Warner Books, 1995

Schmall, PhD, Vicki L., Cleland, RN, Marilyn, Sturdevant, RN, MSW, LCSW, Marilynn *The Caregiver Helpbook, Powerful Tools for Caregiving.* Legacy Health Systems, 2000

Spock, M.D., Benjamin, *Dr. Spock's Baby and Child Care.* Pocket Books Publishing, 1998

Strozzi, Richard *The Anatomy of Change, A Way to Move Through Life's Transitions*, Heckler. North Atlantic Books, 1993

Thomas, *David Improving Your Memory.* DK Publishing, 2003

Tsu, Lao *Tao Te Ching*, translated by Gia-fu Feng & Jane English. NY: Random House, Vantage Books, 1972

Vaillant, MD, George E. *Aging Well*, Little. Brown and Company, 2002

Von Foerster, Heinz, *Understanding Understandings: Essays on Cybernetics and Cognition.* New York: Springer Verlag, 2003

Wade, Carlson *Eat Away Illness.* Parker Publishing Company, 1986

Weil, MD, Andrew, *Healthy Aging.* NY: Alfred A. Knopf, 2006

Winterson, Jeanette, *Oranges Are Not The Only Fruit.* London: Pandora Press, 1985

Zeisel, PhD., John, *I'm Still Here. A Breakthrough Approach to Understanding Someone Living with Alzheimer's.* NY: Penguin Group, 2009

Helpful Resources

AARP, 601 E Street NW, Washington, DC 20049; 202-434-2277; www.aarp.org

AARP Pharmacy Services, Walgreens Health Services, P.O. Box 2301, Muscle Shoals, AL 35662; 800-456-2277; www.aarppharmacy.com

Administration on Aging, One Massachusetts Avenue, Suites 4100 & 5100, Washington, DC 20201; 202-619-0724; www.aoa.dhhs.gov

Aerobics and Fitness Foundation, 15250 Ventura Boulevard, Suite 200, Sherman Oaks, CA 91403; 800-BE-FIT-86; contactafaa@afaa.com

Aging Network Services, Topaz House, 4400 East-West Highway, Bethesda, MD 20814; 301-657-4329; www.agingnets.com

Aging Well (The Magazine for Professionals Promoting Positive Aging), 3801 Schuylkill Road, Spring City, PA 19475; 610-948-9500; www.agingwellmag.com

ALS Association, National Office, 27001 Agoura Road, Suite 250, Calabasas Hills, CA 91301-5104; 818-880-9007; www.alsa.org

Alzheimer's Disease Education Referral Center, Box 8057, Gaithersburg, MD 20898; 800-438-4380; www.nia.nih.gov/alzheimers

American Association of Homes for the Aging, 2519 Connecticut Avenue NW, Washington DC 20008; 202-783-2242; www.aahsa.org

American Cancer Society; 800-227-2345; PO BOX 22718, Oklahoma city, OK 73123-1718; www.cancer.org

American College of Sports Medicine, Dept 6022, Carol Stream, IL 60122-6022; 317-637-9200; www.acsm.org

American Diabetes Association, 1701 N Beauregard Street, Alexandria, VA 22311; 703-549-1500; www.diabetes.org

American Dietetic Association, 120 S Riverside Plaza, Suite 2000, Chicago, IL 60606-6995; 800-877-1600; www.eatright.org

American Foundation for the Blind, 11 Penn Plaza, Suite 300, New York, NY 10001; 212-502-7600; www.afb.org; afbinfo@afb.net

American Geriatrics Society, The Empire State Building, 350 Fifth Avenue, Suite 801, New York, NY 10118; 212-308-1414; www.americangeriatrics.org; info@americangeriatrics.org

American Heart Association, 7272 Greenville Avenue, Dallas, TX 75231; 800-AHA-USA1; www.americanheart.org

American Hospital Association Services, 840 N Lakeshore Drive, Chicago, IL 60611; 800-242-2626; www.aha.org

American Lung Association, 61 Broadway, New York, NY 10006; 212-315-8700; www.lungusa.org

American Medical Association, 515 N State Street, Chicago, IL 60610; 800-621-8335; www.ama-assn.org

American Nurses Association, 8515 Georgia Avenue, Suite 400, Silver Spring, MD 20910-3492; 301-628-5000; www.nursingworld.org

American Parkinson's Disease Association, 135 Parkinson Avenue, Staten Island, NY 10305; 800-223-2732; www.apdaparkinson.org

American Red Cross, 2025 E Street NW, Washington, DC 20006; 703-206-6000; www.redcross.org

American Senior Fitness Association, P.O. Box 2572, New Smyma Beach, FL 32170; 888-689-6791; www.seniorfitness.net

American Society on Aging, 833 Market Street, Suite 511, San Francisco, CA 94103; 415-974-9617; www.asaging.org

Arthritis Foundation, 2970 Peachtree Road NW, Suite 200, Atlanta, GA 30305; 800-283-7800; www.arthritis.org

Better Hearing Institute, 1444 I Street NW, Suite 700, Washington, DC 20005; 202-449-1100; www.betterhearing.org; mail@betterhearing.org

Center for Applied Research on Aging and Health, Home Environmental Assessment Protocol (for Dementia), 130 S 9th Street, Suite 513, Philadelphia, PA 19107; 215-503-4716; www.jefferson.edu/jchp/carah

Center for Healthy Aging, National Council on Aging, 1901 L Street, NW, 4th FL, Washington, DC 20036; 202-479-1200; www.healthyprograms.org

Center for Medicare and Medicaid Services, 7500 Security Boulevard, Baltimore, MD 21224; 800-633-4227; www.cms.hhs.gov

Centers for Disease Control and Prevention, 1600 Clifton Road NE, Atlanta, GA 30330; 800-232-4636; www.cdc.gov

Clinical Trials, A Service of the U.S. National Institutes of Health, 9000 Rockville Pike, Bethesda, MD 20892; 301-496-4000; www.clinicaltrials.gov

Deaf Counseling, Advocacy and Referral Agency, 14895 E 14th Street, Suite 200, San Leandro, CA 94578-2926; 877-322-7288; www.dcara.org; info@dcara.org

Disability Rights Advocates, 2001 Center Street, 4th FL, Berkeley, CA 94704-1204; 510-665-8644; www.dralegal.org; general@dralegal.org

Elder Treks, 597 Markham Street, Toronto, ON M6G 2L7, Canada; 800-741-7956; www.eldertreks.com; adventure@eldertreks.com

Eldercare Locator, 1700 Rhode Island Avenue NW, Suite 1200, Washington DC 20036; 800-677-1116; www.eldercare.gov

Elderhostel, 11 Avenue de Lafayette, Boston, MA 02111; 800-454-5768; www.elderhostel.org

Fall Prevention Center of Excellence, University of Southern California Andrus Gerontology Center, 3715 McClintock Avenue, Room

228, Los Angeles, CA 90089-0191; 213-740-7069; www.stopfalls.org; info@stopfalls.org

Family Caregiver Alliance, 180 Montgomery Street, Suite 1100, San Francisco, CA 94104; 415-434-3388; www.caregiver.org

Food and Nutrition Information Center, National Agricultural Library, 10301 Baltimore Avenue, Room 105, Beltsville, MD 20705; 301-504-5414

Gerontological Society of America, 1220 L Street NW, Suite 901, Washington DC 20005; 202-854-1275; www.geron.org

Housing Enabler, Susanne Iwarsson, Professor, Occupational Therapist, Veten & Skapen HB, Pl 2532, SE 28893 Navlinge, Sweden; 46-46-222 19 40; www.enabler.nu; susanne.iwarsson@med.lu.se

Lab Tests Online (A guide to understanding lab test results), AACC, 1850 K Street NW, Suite 625, Washington, DC 20006; www.labtestsonline.org

Lifelong Fitness Alliance, 658 Bair Island Road, Suite 200, Redwood City, CA 94063; 650-361-8282; www.50plus.org

Logisticare (Medicaid transportation); 1800 Phoenix Blvd., Suite 120, Atlanta, Georgia; 1-800-486-7647; www.logisticare.com,

Lumetra (Independent Medical Reviewers-Medicare), One Sansome Street, San Francisco, CA 94104; 800-841-1602; www.lumetra.com; info@lumetra.com

Meals on Wheels Association of America, 203 S Union Street, Alexandria, VA 22314; 703-548-5558; www.mowaa.org; mowaa@mowaa.org

Medicare, Centers for Medicare & Medicaid Services, 7500 Security Boulevard, Baltimore, MD 21244-1850; 800-633-4227; www.medicare.gov

National Aging in Place Council, 1400 16th Street NW, Suite 420, Washington, DC 20036; 202-939-1784; www.naipc.org/naipchome/tabid/36/default.aspx

National Alliance of Senior Citizens, Peter Luciano, 2525 Wilson Boulevard, Arlington, VA 22201; www.health.gov/nhic

National Association for Home Care & Hospice, 228 Seventh Street SE, Washington, DC 20003; 202-547-7424; www.nahc.org

National Association of Area Agencies on Aging (n4a), 1730 Rhode Island Avenue NW, Suite 1200, Washington, DC 20036; 202-872-0888; www.n4a.org

National Cancer Institute, Public Inquiries Office, 6116 Executive Boulevard, Room 3036A, Bethesda, MD 20892-8322; 800-422-6237; www.cancer.gov; cancergovstaff@mail.nih.gov

National Capital Poison Center, 1220 L Street NW, Suite 800, Washington, DC 20005; 202-637-8400; www.poison.org; pc@poison.org

National Caucus and Center on Black Aged, Inc., 1220 L Street NW, Suite 800, Washington, DC 20005; 202-637-8400; www.ncba-aged.org

National Center for Injury Prevention and Control, Mailstop K65, 4770 Buford Highway NE, Atlanta, GA 30341-3724; 800-232-4636; http://www.cdc.gov/ncipc/pub-res/toolkit/CheckListForSafety.htm

National Center on Elder Abuse, c/o Center for Community Research and Services, University of Delaware, 297 Graham Hall, Newark, DE 19716; 302-831-3525; www.ncea.aoa.gov

National Center on Senior Transportation, 1425 K Street NW, Suite 200, Washington, DC 20005; 866-528-NCST; www.seniortransportation.net

National Citizens Coalition for Nursing Home Reform (NCCNHR), 1828 L Street NW, Suite 801, Washington, DC 20036; 202-332-2276; www.nccnhr.org

National Council on Aging, 1901 L Street NW, 4th FL, Washington, DC 20036; 202-479-1200; www.ncoa.org; info@ncoa.org

National Council on Alcoholism and Drug Dependence, Inc., 244 E 58th Street, 4th FL, New York, NY 10022; 212-269-7797; www.ncadd.org; national@ncadd.org

National Eye Institute, Information Office, 31 Center Drive, MSC 2510, Bethesda, MD 20892-2510; 301-496-5248; www.nei.nih.gov; 2020@nei.nih.gov

National Guideline Clearinghouse (for Health Conditions); www.guideline.gov

National Heart Lung and Blood Institute, NHLBI Health Information Center, PO Box 30105, Bethesda, MD 20824-0105; 301-592-8573; www.nhlbi.nih.gov; nhlbiinfo@nhlbi.nih.gov

National Hospice & Palliative Care Organization, 1700 Diagonal Road, Suite 625, Alexandria, VA 22314; 703-837-1500; www.nhpco.org; nhpco_info@nhpco.org

National Immunization Hotline, Centers for Disease Control & Prevention, 1600 Clifton Road NE, Atlanta, GA 30330; 800-232-4636; www.cdc.gov/vaccines/

National Institute of Arthritis and Musculoskeletal and Skin Diseases (NIAMS), Information Clearinghouse, National Institutes of Health, 1 AMS Circle, Bethesda, MD 20892-3675; 877-226-4267; www.niams.nih.gov; NIAMSinfo@mail.nih.gov

National Institute of Neurological Disorders and Stroke, NIH Neurological Institute, P.O. Box 5801, Bethesda, MD 20824; 800-352-9424; www.ninds.nih.gov

National Institute on Aging, Building 31, Room 5C27, 31 Center Drive, MSC 2292, Bethesda, MD 20892; 301-496-1752; www.nia.nih.gov

National Institute on Deafness and Other Communication Disorders, Information Office, Building 31, Room 3C35, 9000 Rockville Pike, Bethesda, MD 20852; 301-496-7243; www.nih.gov

National Legal Aid & Defender Association, 1140 Connecticut Avenue NW, Suite 900, Washington, DC 20036; 202-452-0620; www.nlada.org

National Long Term Care Ombudsman Resource Center, ORC Office, 1828 L Street NW, Suite 801, Washington, DC 20036; 202-332-2275; www.ltcombudsman.org; ombudcenter@nccnhr.org

National Mental Health Association, Mental Health America, 2000 N Beauregard Street, 6th FL, Alexandria, VA 22311; 800-969-6642; www.nmha.org

National Multiple Sclerosis Society, 1800 M Street NW, Suite 750 South, Washington, DC 20036; 800-344-4867; www.nationalmssociety.org

National Osteoporosis Foundation, 1232 22nd Street NW, Washington, DC 20037-1202; 800-231-4222; www.nof.org

National Rehabilitation Information Center, 8201 Corporate Drive, Suite 600, Landover, MD 20785; 800-346-2742; www.naric.com

National Senior Citizens Education and Research Center, Inc., 8403 Colesville Road, Silver Spring, MD 20910; 301-578-8510

National Senior Citizens Law Center, 1444 Eye Street NW, Suite 1100, Washington, DC 20005; 202-289-6976; www.nscatogether.org/about.us.htm

National Stroke Association, 9707 E Easter Lane, Building B, Centennial, CO 80112; 800-787-6537; www.stroke.org

Nursing Home Information Service, National Council of Senior Citizens Education and Research Center, Centers for Medicare & Medicaid Services, 7500 Security Boulevard, Baltimore, MD 21244-1850; 800-633-4227; www.medicare.gov/Nursing/Overview.asp

Parkinson's Disease Foundation, 1359 Broadway, Suite 1509, New York, NY 10018; 212-923-4700; www.pdf.org; info@pdf.org

Philips Lifeline, Home Safety Monitors, Philips Healthcare, 3000 Minuteman Road, Andover, MA 01810-1099; 800-934-7372; www.lifelinesys.com

President's Council on Physical Fitness and Sports, Department W, 200 Independence Avenue SW, Room 738-H, Washington, DC 20201-0004; 202-690-9000; www.fitness.gov

Prevent Blindness America, 211 West Wacker Drive, Suite 1700, Chicago, IL 60606; 800-331-2020; www.preventblindness.org

Senior Corps, 1201 New York Avenue NW, Washington, DC 20525; 202-606-5000; www.seniorcorps.org

Senior Net, 900 Lafayette Street, Suite 604, Santa Clara, CA 95050; 408-615-0699; www.seniornet.org

Senior Service America, 8403 Colesville Road, Suite 1200, Silver Spring, MD 20910; 301-578-8900; www.seniorserviceamerica.org; contact@ssa-I.org

Senior Ventures , Siskiyou Center, South Oregon University, 1250 Boulevard, Cox Hall, Ashland, OR 97520; 800-257-0577; www.sou.edu/siskiyoucenter/seniorventures

Service Corps of Retired Executives (SCORE Association), 409 3rd Street SW, 6th FL, Washington, DC 20024; 800-634-0245; www.score.org

Social Security Administration, Office of Public Inquiries, Windsor Park Building, 6401 Security Boulevard, Baltimore, MD 21235; 800-772-1213; www.socialsecurity.gov

Soundbytes (Independent Hearing Products), P.O. Box 9022, Hicksville, NY 11802; 888-816-8191; www.soundbytes.com

Substance Abuse & Mental Health Services Administration, SAMHSA's Health Information Network, P.O. Box 2345, Rockville, MD 20847-2345; 877-726-4727; www.samhsa.gov/shin; SHIN@samhsa.hhs.gov

U.S. Department of Health and Human Services, Office of Disease Prevention and Health Promotion, 200 Independence Avenue SW, Washington, DC 20201; 877-696-6775; www.hhs.gov

U.S. Department of Labor Employee Benefits Security Administration, Frances Perkins Building, 200 Constitution Avenue NW, Washington, DC 20210; 866-444-EBSA; www.dol.gov/ebsa

U.S. Department of Health and Human Services, Office of Disease Prevention and Health Promotion, Office of Public Health and Science, Office of the Secretary, 1101 Wootton Parkway, Suite LL100, Rockville, MD 20852; 240-453-8280; http://odphp.osophs.dhhs.gov

U.S. Food and Drug Administration, 5600 Fishers Lane, Rockville, MD 20857; 888-463-6332; www.fda.gov

USDA Meat & Poultry Hotline; 888-674-6854; www.fsis.usda.gov; mphotline.fsis@usda.gov

Vestibular Disorders Association, P.O. Box 13305, Portland, OR 97213-0305; 800-837-8428; www.vestibular.org

Visiting Nurse Associations of America, 900 19th Street NW, Suite 200, Washington, DC 20006; 202-384-1420; www.vnaa.org; vnaa@vnaa.org

Index

Photographs are marked by *italic* "*ph*" and page number. Example: David (Cousin), *34ph*

Illustrations are marked by *italic* "*Ill*" and page number. Example: brain, the, and memory, *74ill*

A
"a nurse with a purse," 151
a priori, 258
acceptance
 of aging, 214, 243–245
 of alternative treatments, 114, 118
 of humor in adversity, 10
 phase of memory loss, 62, 66
 and self-actualization, 248
 in stages of dying, 183–184
 of transitions, 5
acronyms, 102, 272–273
action plan, 172–174
"Active for Life," exercise program, 121
active listening, 197–198
acupuncture, 114, 115–117, 257
 see also auriculotherapy
acute diseases, 82
Adams, Scott, 179
ADD (Attention Deficit Disorder), 59–60, 257
ADL (Activities of Daily Living), 257
 caregiver performs, 72
Adult Day Health Center, 65, 225, 257
adversity
 factors affecting, 81
 perseverance and, 128
 seeing through, 166–167
 staying positive during, 46, 99–101
 transcending, 200
 use of humor and, 10, 205
agape, 131, 257
aging, 215
 baby boomers, 37, 39, 106, 258
 and change, 43–49
 and chronic disease, 79–83 (*See also* chronic diseases)
 and creativity, 83–87
 definition of, 257
 healthy, 105–112, 120, 278, 281
 making peace with, 243–246
 memory loss with, 50–55, 73–75, *74ill*
 normal, 75–76
 paradigm, 7–9, *9ill*
 in place, 217–220
 plight of, 4–11
 and realizing potential, 209–216
 study of, 264
 ugliness of, 234
aging process
 aspects of, 243–246, 253–254
 change and, 42
 chronic disease accelerating, 99–101
 disease as dynamic in, 81
 Fountain of Youth, 80, 92, 128, 235, 263
 as a gift, 42
 handling challenges of, 164
 making peace with, 80, 212, 218
 memory loss associated with, 90
 nurturing, 92
agnosia, 257
agreement, 144, 159–160, 170, 173
AIDS (Acquired Immune Deficiency Syndrome), 257
 See also HIV (Human Immunodeficiency Virus)
Akiva, Rabbi, ix
Albom, Mitch

289

Tuesdays with Morrie, 205
alcohol use, 75, 83, 89, 102, 110, 119
Allen, Fred, 174
Allen, Woody, 181, 237
alternative medicine, 114–129
   acupuncture, 114, 115–116, 117, 257
   auriculotherapy, 258
   chiropractic care, 114, 116–119, 259
   exercise and diet, 120–128
Alzheimer's disease
   causing memory loss, 77
   definition of, 257
   diagnosis of, 88–90
   drug therapy for, 53
   free radicals and, 263
   hospice care and, 203
   intimacy and, 149–150
   staving off, 211
   testing for, 57–58
American College of Sports Medicine, 124
amygdala, 75
Anatomy of an Illness as Perceived by the Patient (Cousins), 10–11
anesthesia, 258
anger
   and Alzheimer's disease, 57–58
   and healthy family dynamics, 175
   as part of stages of dying, 183, 185
antioxidants, 91, 103
antismoking bill, 83
anxiety
   about forming relationships, 135, 143, 153, 154
   about pain, 10
   crisis and, 162–163, *163ill*, 164–165, 167
   grieving and, 188, 197–198
   memory loss and, 102
   selfish acts and, 169
   visualizations to treat, 114
aphasia (language problems), 88, 258
apraxia, 258
archeologist, 258

Aricept (Donepezil), drug, 53
Art of Happiness (Dalai Lama), 236–237, 277
arteries, 61, 88, 122
arthritis
   definition of, 258
   and drug interactions, 44
   juvenile rheumatoid, 97
   noninvasive treatments for, 117
   osteo-, 97
   rheumatoid, 85, 96–98, 263, 267, 271
Ashkenazi Jews, 58, 258
assisted living, 68, 154–155, 177, 195, 206, 258
associations, making, 77
asthma, 116–117
attachment, 47, 231
attachment disorder, 230, 233, 258
attitude
   adapting to memory loss and, 66, 78
   definition of, 258
   good, in old age, 214
   happiness and, 224, 238
   heart disease and, 12
   impact of, 184
   maintaining humanitarian, 226
   positive, 101
   in process of change, 48
   stress and, 47
auriculotherapy, 258
   see also acupuncture
autoimmune disease, 96, 258
autonomic nervous system, 260, 265, 268
autonomous will, 41
average life-span, 11, 83, 96, 109, 245

B
Babe, Ruth, 129
baby boomers, 37, 39, 106, 244, 258
background checks, for caregiver, 71
bandwagon, 258
bargaining, 183–184
behavioral therapy, 102

benchmarks, 33, 109, 128, 169, 258
benevolence, 16
beta-carotene, 91
Better Business Bureau, 73
birthing process, 41–42
black outs, 52
black sheep, 170, 171
Blake, Eubie, 83
blindness, 96
blood
  cells, white, 266
  clots, 61
  fluids, 122
  pressure, 110, 112, 117, 134, 135, 260
  sugar, 260
  thinners, 103, 115, 260
Bloomfield, Harold H.
  Making Peace with your Parents, 185
bonded, Home Health Agencies, 73, 259
"boomer triangle," 244
boomers, 37, 39, 106, 258
Bortz, Walter, 12
  Dare To Be 100, 109
Botox, 244
Boy Scout Motto, x
BRACA 1/BRACA 2 genes, 58
brain, the
  and Alzheimer's disease, 77, 88, 90, 257
  aneurysms, 61–62
  cells, 51, 74, 77
  as computer, 87
  definition of, 51
  and habits, 111
  and happiness, 224
  and memory, 73–75, *74ill*
  mental stimulation of, 65, 102, 103
  mental "tapes" of, 162
  and physical activity, 212, 221
  pleasure centers of, 144
  speech center of, 86
  spotting, 76
  Tau protein in, 53

brain-dead, 182
brainstorming, 173
breadwinner, 112, 259
breathing
  and asthma, 117
  controlled, 49, 113
  with partner, 143–144
Bridges, William, 47
  Transitions, 36
Britt, Lucille, 181
Brompton's cocktail, 202
Broudy, Joe (Uncle), *28ph*, *34ph*
Broudy, Leah (Aunt), 26–27, *28ph*, *34ph*
brushing teeth, 96, 97, 109
  See also teeth
Bubbie, definition of, 259
Bubbie (Paternal Grandmother), *11ph*, 17–18, *34ph*
Buck Institute for Geriatric Research (Marin County, CA), 53
The Bucket List (movie), 254
Buddhist religion, 47, 217
Burns, George, 10, 244
bushman, living like, 109, 259
butterflies, 220, 221, 267

C

calendars, keeping, 77, 101
California (CA), Buck Institute for Geriatric Research, 53
Callanan, Maggie
  Final Gifts, 197
cancer
  colon, 58, 203–204
  definition of, 259
  free radicals and, 263
  genetic testing for, 58–59
  hospice care and, 203
  lung, 183
  multiple myelona, 93
  prostate, 91
  quality time and, 165
carbohydrates, 12, 123–
cardiac arrest, 98

cardiovascular disease, 83, 259
cards, playing, 102
caregivers
　definition of, 259
　family members as, 164, 165
　intimacy and, 142–144, 145, 147
　for memory impaired person, 68–71, 100–102
　screening of, 61–62, 71–73
caressing, 143, 145, 147
Carroll, Lewis, 1
Carter, Jimmy
　Virtues of Aging, The, 251
Casals, Pablo, 85
CAT scan, 88, 90
　See also CT scan
Catholic faith wake, 189
celebrations, 189–190, 196, 207, 261
cells
　brain, 51, 74, 77, 212
　cancer, 259
　diabetes, 261
　genes and, 263
　preservation of, 271
　protoplasm, 270
　repair of, 91
　serum and blood, 122, 266
　white blood, 266
centenarians, 259
Centers for Disease Control (CDC), 134, 284
cephalopodan, 51, 259
cerebral cortex, 74, 74*ill*, 86, 259
certifications, of caregiver, 72
Chamber Of Commerce, 73
changes
　aging, 43–49
　of, 259
　loss, 66–67
　making, 168–

chess, 102
Chi, 259
child, inner, 4, 33, 41–42, 48, 128, 246, 255
Childs, George Williams, 142
China, ix
　medicine in, 115–116, 117
　word meaning crisis, 165
chiropractic care, 114, 116–119, 259
chocolate, 128, 224
choices
　being alone and, 152, 228
　conscious, 44
　as essence of living, 220
　freedom to make, 230
　happiness and, 229
　making, 36, 38
　planning analyses for making, 168–169, 174–175
　promoting guilt, 206
　taking responsibility for, 159
cholesterol, 122
cholinesterase inhibitors, 53, 90, 104, 259
Christian faith, wake, 189
chronic diseases, 92–102
　aging and, 79–83, 99–101, 244
　and challenging oneself, 101
　definition of, 260
　edentulousness related to, 96
　melanoma removal, 94–95
　multiple myeloma, 93
　osteoarthritis as, 97
　of partners, 142–143
　periodontal disease related to, 95–96
　statistics on, 125
　See also individual diseases
chronic obstructive pulmonary disease (COPD), 203, 228, 260
chrysalis, 42, 260
Churchill, Sir Winston, 179
circle of compassion, 228
coffins, 187, 196
Cognex (Tacrine), drug, 53
cognition, 260

cognitive
  impairments, 172
  problems, 53
  testing, 59
cognitive impairment, mild (MCI), 76, 90–91, 268
colon cancers, 58, 203–204
colonoscopy, 203, 260
coming of age, 6
communication, 153–154, 155, 159, 170, 197
communication style, of caregiver, 72
companions, 151–152, 248
companionship, 133, 140
compassion, 89, 227, 228
concentration camps, 17, 45–46
conservators, 69
consistency in care, for memory impaired person, 65–66, 73
control, 107, 132, 188, 193, 197, 230
COPD (chronic obstructive pulmonary disease), 203, 228, 260
corporate like meetings, 63, 65, 170–171, 260
cortisol, 112, 260
cost-of-living raises, for caretaker, 73
Coumadin, drug, 115, 260
counseling
  about a disease, 206, 213
  about isolation, 229, 233
  about sex, 135
  for bad sexual experience, 132
  for children, 191
  elders, 56, 214, 231
  in exercise programs, 121
  to help family member in crisis, *163ill*, 172
  in life crisis, 2–3
  as mental conditioning, 108
  with partner, 135
Cousins, Norman, 84–85
  Anatomy of an Illness as Perceived by the Patient, 10–11
CPR (cardiopulmonary resuscitation)
  definition of, 260

training, 71
creativity, 66, 83–87, 225, 248, 260
crisis
  during changes, 37
  counseling, 2, 172
  definition of, 165
  determining what is best for parent, 62
  due to unmet needs, 179
  in families, 62, 66, 162–163, *163ill*, 164–169, 174–176
  families experience, 164
  financial, 234–235
  from financial loss, 3
  planning in families, 174–176
criticism, 118, 251
crossword puzzles, 102, 212
CT scan, 53, 260
  See also CAT scan
cultivating relationships, 215–216
CVA (cerebral vascular accident), 61, 260
cycles, life, 42

D

Dalai Lama, His Holiness the, 41, 222, 260
  Art of Happiness, 236–237, 277
dancing, 102, 103, 157–158, 211
Danny (Cousin), 31, *34ph*
Dare To Be 100 (Bortz), 109
dating services, 137–139
David (Cousin), 31, *34ph*
Days of the Dead, The (Los Dias de las Muertes), 189–190, 261
De Angelis, Barbara, 157
death, 180–202
  after life, 217
  average age at, 11, 83
  celebrations around, 189–190, 196, 207, 261
  definition of, 182
  documents in preparation of, important, 193–196
  and dying, 181–187

and emotions, 190–191, 197
family preparation for a, 165
and finding route of self-discovery, 198–200
funeral custom, 188, 190, 196
and grieving process, 188–191, 198, 200–201
hospice care, as part of process of, 202–207, 265
legal documents in preparation of, 69, 178, 193, 195–196, 261, 270, 273, 274
opening communications about, 197–198
of parents, 185–187
See also dying process
decision-making process, 48, 174
dehydration, 52, 260
delusions, 260, 271
dementia
causing memory loss, 76–77
definition of, 261
drug therapy for, 53
effects of, 22–23
of elderly, 88–90
and erectile dysfunction, 134
help with memory, 102–104
and intimacy, 148–149
and mild cognitive impairment, 268
people perceptions of, 248–250
and response to crisis, 168
selenium for treating, 91
wandering and, 92, 104
See also Alzheimer's disease
dementia praecox, 271
denial, 57, 66, 181, 183, 219
dental hygiene *See* teeth
Department of Health and Human Services, 286
depersonalization, 187, 204
depression
aging as cause for, 45, 76
and being a victim, 230
and being alone, 226
causing memory loss, 76

and change, 36, 46
definition of, 261
and erectile dysfunction, 134
and helping others, 46
and humor, 10
from medications, 44–45
as part of stages of dying, 183
from a physical loss, 2–3
and satisfaction, 224–225
and stress, 76
dextrose, 123–124
diabesity, 124
diabetes, 83, 96, 124, 134, 228, 261
Diane (Cousin), 29
diary *See* journaling
Dias de las Muertes, Los (The Days of the Dead), 189–190, 261
diets
deficiencies, causing memory loss, 76
and exercise, 120–128
and longevity, 12
poor, 83
proper, 12, 15, 83, 102, 109, 123
to treat MCI, 91
See also eating
digestive tract, 96, 261
dignity
dying with, 189, 204
keeping ones, 110
as keys to happiness, 226, 228–231, 238–241
definition of, 6, 261
disabilities, 3, 72, 96, 125, 261
Disc Analysis, 72
diseases
autoimmune, 258
cardiovascular, 83, 259
heart, 11–12, 96, 119, 263
kidney, 52
lung, 54, 82, 272
pancreatic, 261
periodontal, 82–83, 95–96
systemic, 76, 82, 83, 271, 272
understanding, 79–82
See also individual diseases

divorces, 95, 138, 150–151, 160
documents
  important, 193–196
  legal, 69, 178, 193, 195–196, 261, 270, 273, 274
Dolphin Running Club, San Francisco, 110
Don Quixote, 160, 261
Donepezil (Aricept), drug, 53
dopamine, 111, 269
dreams, 130, 142, 158, 222–223, 225
drinking
  alcohol, 75, 83, 89, 102, 110, 119
  water, 51, 109
drinking fluids, 51
drivers license, of caregiver, 71–72
drugs
  and aging, 99
  causing memory loss, 75
  delivering, 104
  for dementia, 53, 164
  for erectile dysfunction, 97, 134–135, 262, 273
  and hypnosis, 115
  illicit use of, 83, 111, 204, 268
  interaction of, 44–45, 261
  L-Dopa, 98
  precautions using, 110
durable power of healthcare, 193, 261
Dutch, the, and heart disease, 119
dying process
  aging and, 243 (*See also* death)
  funeral preparations as part of, 196
  hospice care and, 197, 207
  leaving a legacy, 191–192
  maintaining dignity during, 189
  making peace with, 185
  reactions to, 6–7, 182
  rebirth and, 205
  sharing feelings and thoughts during, 198
dying with dignity, 189, 204
Dylan, Bob, 238

E

Easwaran, Eknath, 211
eating
  and happiness, 224, 235
  right, 12, 15, 83, 102, 109, 123
  See also diets
economist, 262
ED (erectile dysfunction), 97, 134–135, 262, 273
edentulousness, 96
Edie (Cousin), 31, *34ph*
Edison, Charles, 166–167
Edison, Thomas, 166–167, 273
Edwards, Jennifer, 208
E-harmony.com, dating service, 137
e-heath, 262
Ehrmann, Max, 79
Einstein, Albert, 227–228, 273
Eisenhower, Dwight David, 177
elders
  challenging the brain of, 220–221
  with compromised loved ones, 142
  definition of, 262
  facing chronic disease and, 101
  getting in touch with inner child, 128, 207
  internal changes in, 48
  learning new technology, 39
  listening to, 13
  mild cognitive impairment and, 90–91
  relationships with, 18–21
  sexually transmitted diseases and, 97
  in skilled nursing facilities, 23
  in society, 7
  transitioning to, 23
  volunteering to help others, 220
EMDR treatment modality, for PTSD, 76
emotional pain, 181, 185–187, 190, 198, 200–202, 206–207
emotions
  acting out of, 164
  and death, 197
  during grieving process, 190–191

and hippocampus, 75
and negativity, 224–225
empathic, 43, 72, 262
emphysema, 82, 85
Enbrel, drug, 97–98
endocrine, 261–262, 269
endorphins, 111, 113, 144, 224–225, 238, 262
energy
  and bad relationships, 154
  channels, 115, 257, 267
  from chocolate, 128
  and exercise, 122
  from intimacy, 132
  renewal, 112–113
  from shared love, 205
enlightenment, 47, 109
enzymes, 89, 122–124, 259, 263, 271
epinephrine, 112, 113
epiphany, 2, 254, 262
erectile dysfunction (ED), 97, 134–135, 262, 273
Erickson, Erik, 6, 41–42
evolutionary changes, 38
executive dysfunction, 262
Exelon (Rivastigmine), drug, 53
exercise
  of brain, 65, 102, 103
  and cardiac output, 110
  in counseling program, 121
  and diet, 122–125, 128
  and energy, 111, 122
  gurus, 106
  as a habit, 111
  and longevity, 12–13
  and Parkinson's disease, 98–99
  as part of mental conditioning, 102
  regular, 83, 102, 109, 120–123, 126–127
  and strokes, 87
eyesight impairment, 96

F

facilities
  Adult Day Health Center, 257
  assisted-living, 154–155, 177, 195, 206, 258
  in China, 116
  for memory impaired, 89, 92, 104
  skilled nursing, 23, 80, 195, 202
family
  caretakers, 73
  crisis, 62, 66, 162–169, *163ill*, 174–176
  during dying process, 203–207
  dynamics, 23, 33, 66, 169, 171–173, 175, 193
  history, 13, 16–17, 20, 22–23
  maps, 38, 263
  principles, 31–32
  transitions, 167–171, 176–179
fatal diseases, 82
fats, trans, 12, 122–124
fatty acids, 91
  free, 122–123
fear
  of being alone, 226
  of cancer, 203
  causing cognitive problems, 52–53
  of death, 188, 197, 207
  definition of, 263
  in forming relationships, 132, 135, 142, 143, 154
  and memory loss, 55, 57
  uncovering, 46
  of unknown, 118, 173, 181, 231
Fields, W. C., 120, 221
Final Gifts (Callanan), 197
Finesilver, Sherman, 129
First Law of Evolving System Dynamics, 173, 274
first-aid training, for caregiver, 72
flax seed, 91
flexibility of caregiver, 72
flossing teeth, 96, 97, 109
  See also teeth
food *See* diets
Ford, Henry, 141
foreign caregivers, 68–69
foreplay, 144, 145, 263

Fountain of Youth, 80, 92, 128, 235, 263
four noble truths, 47
France, and heart disease, 119
Frankl, Victor
   Man's Search for Meaning, 45–46, 199
Franny (Aunt), 28–31
Franz Josef I (Emperor of Austria), 19–20
free fatty acids, 122–123
free radicals, 263
Freud, Clement, 110
Frost, Robert, 155
   Road Not Taken, 35–36
Frye, Mary Elizabeth, 187
functional impairments, 88
funerals, 188, 190, 196

G

Galantamine (Reminyl), drug, 53
Gandhi, Mahatma, 107, 230
Gates, Bill, 136–137
Gene (case study), living with cancer, 212–214
generic drugs for memory loss therapy, 53
genes, 58, 88–89, 263
genetic testing, 57–58, 88–89
genetics, 11, 51, 59, 111–112, 125, 214
genograms (family maps), 38, 263
Georgia (case study), in finding meaning, 46–47
geriatricians, 12, 59, 109, 263
gerontologists
   cognitive testing by, 59
   crisis management by, 164, 169–170, 173
   definition of, 264
   managing medications by, 66
   safety evaluation by, 103
gerontology, 3, 116, 264
Gibran, Kahil, 32–33
gifts, the seven, 241–242
ginkgo biloba, 103

Gladys (case study), as victim, 232–233
global positioning system (GPS) devices, 93
goals
   achieving, 95
   of happiness, 227
   long-term, 174–175
   personal, 172
   for relationships, 156
   setting, 3, 33, 109, 167–169, 173, 174–175
   short-term, 174–175, 177
GPS (global positioning system) devices, 93, 264
grace, 5–6
grandmothers, Jewish, 259, 268
grass roots, 264
Greer (case study), on aging and creativity, 84
grief, 264
grieving
   a death, 185–191, 198, 200–201
   a physical loss, 2–3
   process, 188–191
   and transcendence, 199–200
group therapy, 135
guided imagery, 112, 114, 190–191, 264
guilt
   and coming close to death, 197
   from discovering a lie, 249
   disrupting family dynamic, 169
   moving on without, 154
   promoting mental angst, 206, 229
   and punishing yourself, 199–200
gum disease, 82–83, 95–96
gurus, 106, 264

H

Hanh, Thich Nhat, 49
happiness
   benefits of, 107
   books about happiness, 237
   choice as a role in, 229
   definition of, 225

ebbs and flows of, 37
emotional, 250–251
finding, 225–226
finding place in crisis, restoring, 172
from helping others, 13
intimacy and, 146
introspection as tool for, 227
keys to, 226, 228–231, 238–241
maintaining, 234–241
quest for, 37
self–sufficiency and, 231
state of, 222, 223–225, 237
true, 47
ultimate, 221, 253
happyness (purposeful misspelling), 225, 264
harmony, 107, 113, 115, 207, 259
Harriet (case study), on memory loss, 52–54
Harry (Second Cousin) "the old man," 15–16, 23
Harvard University, 109
Hawthorne, Nathaniel, 221
Hayes, Helen, 204–205
head injuies, causing memory loss, 76
healing
    and aging, 82
    the brain, 87
    and Chinese medicine, 115–116, 117
    creating internal environment of, 93
    in family crisis, 62
    and forgiveness, 201
    and grieving process, 185, 190–191
    with others, 198
    and a positive attitude, 108
    power of humor, 10
    process, 3, 188, 196
    through helping others, 189
    trauma of stress, 76
health checks, regular, 101
healthy
    aging, 105–112, 120–128
    family dynamics, 175 (*See also* family: dynamics)
    life, 12, 83, 123

mind, 113
sex, 176
hearing loss, 96
heart
    attacks, 119, 135, 193, 260
    and chocolate, 128
    disease, 96, 120, 203, 263
    and erectile dysfunction, 134–135
    and exercise, 120, 127
Heart To Heart (Swindoll), 48
Heavlin, Noreen Cooper, viii
helping ourselves, 247
Hepatitis B and C, 139
herpes, causing memory loss, 76
hierarchy of needs, 247, 267
    See also Maslow, Abraham
hippocampus, *74ill*, 74–75, 264
history
    family, 13, 16–17, 20, 22–23
    life, 196
    personal, 38, 253
HIV (Human Immunodeficiency Virus), 76, 96–97, 134, 139, 264
    See also AIDS (Acquired Immune Deficiency Syndrome)
holistic/psychological approach, to suffering, 202
Holocaust, 17, 45–46
holographic wills, 194
Home Health Agencies, 68, 71, 73, 264
Home Health Aids, certified, 68, 71
homeopathic alternatives, 114
homeostasis, 248, 265
hormones, 51
    definition of, 265
    endocrine, 144, 262
    pituitary, 269
    PMS and, 270
    steroids and, 112, 113, 272
hospice care, 202–207, 265
"house," in facility, 89
hugging, 103, 109, 143, 144, 145, 146, 224
human nature, 22, 214, 216–219
humanitarian, 265

humor (laughter)
  and ADD behavior, 60
  in fighting disease, 10–11
  and memory loss situations, 57, 78
  sense of, 109, 127, 214–215
  using to break tension, 219–220
Hurwiz, Leonid, 10
hygiene, personal, of caregiver, 72
hypertrophy, 97, 265
hypnosis, 114, 115, 264, 265
hypothalamus, 265

I

I Am Alone (poem) (Shapira), 67
I Am (poem) (Shapira), 201–202
ICU (intensive care unit), 265
identity
  aging with, 11–17
  experiences and, 22
  life direction and, 33
  losing, 1–4
  from personal history, 253
illness
  acceptance of, 185
  associated with stress, 45
  and feelings, 147
  and laughter, 10
  life threatening, 203
  surviving, 108
  and systemic disease, 82
  triaging patients to treat, 202
immortal, 181, 266
immune system, 93, 258, 266
impairments, 76, 88, 90, 108, 172, 266
impermanence, 47
independent contractor, 266
infarct, 266
infections, 76, 204, 266
initiative, isense of, 41
inner child, 4, 33, 41–42, 48, 128, 246, 255
inner self, 46, 142, 199
inner strength, 6, 42, 230, 246
insured, Home Health Agencies, 73
internal changes, 47–48

internal transformation, 40
Internet
  dating services on, 136–139
  medical information on, 119, 134, 262
intimacy, 12, 103, 130–133, 142–150, 266
introspection, as tool for happiness, 227
Italy, and heart disease, 119

J

Japan, and heart disease, 119
J-Date.com, dating service, 137
Jewish Community Centers, 127
Jewish grandmothers, names for, 259, 268
Jewish Home for the Aged (Pittsburgh), 18
Jewish Shivah, 189
Jo (Mother-in-law), 86–87, 151
jobs
  changing, 36–37, 40
  ideal, 211
  and inner transformation, 41
joints
  deformities of, 271
  manipulation of, 116–117
  spinal column, 259
  swelling of, 258
journaling, 77, 102, 185–186, 196
journals, of daily activities, 77
journey, 157, 177, 204, 247, 266
JR (juvenile rheumatoid arthritis), 97
juvenile rheumatoid arthritis (JR), 97

K

Keller, Helen, 95
Khayyam, Omar, 182
kidney disease, 52
kissing, 136, 145, 146
knowledge
  and aging, 7, 34, 211, 215, 243
  and assessing memory loss, 54–55, 62
  and cognition, 260
  gift of, 253

of hospice, 207
of life, 226
need for, 31
of self, 221
and wisdom, 219, 274
Kübler-Ross, Elizabeth, 182–183, 240

L

Language of Feelings, *163ill*
Lao Tzu, 57, 175–176, 216
laughter See humor (laughter)
L-Dopa drugs, 98
Leakey, Richard, 38
learning poems, 102
Lee, Laurie, 150
legacy, 191–192, 251, 253, 266
legal documents, 69, 178, 193, 195–196, 261, 270, 273, 274
LeGette, Marilyn, vii
LeShan, Eda, 152
leukemia, 8, 266, 267
licenses, of caregiver, 69, 72
life
  as change, 40
  complacency in, 138–139
  cycles, 42, 99
  history, 196
  as a process, 95
  purpose in, 84–85
  as suffering, 47
  values, and relationships, 156
life-span, 11, 83, 96, 109, 245
lifestyle
  balanced, 83, 86
  independent, 124–125
  and longevity, 11
  sedentary, 126
lifting requirements, for caregiver, 72
listening, ix, 13, 95, 143–144, 154–155, 197–198
lists, keeping, 77, 102
localized diseases, 82
Loch Ness, Scotland, 225, 266
London, Jack, 196–197, 219
longevity

and creativity, 83–87, 216
definition of, 266
diseases affecting, 83
factors tied to, 11–13, 122, 125, 211
and selenium, 271
in women, 111–112
long-term goals, 174–175
long-term relationships, 140, 150
love
  deep form of love, 131, 257
  entity of, 160
  and the Internet, 136–138
  and intimacy, 131–132
  of self, 110, 148, 160–161, 240, 247–248
  sex as expression of, 144–146
  shared, 205, 207
  true, 150–155
  what you do, 128
lungs, diseases of, 54, 82, 272

M

Macy, R. H., 129
Making Peace with your Parents (Bloomfield), 185
Man's Search for Meaning (Frankl), 45–46, 199
Margulies, Nancy, viii
marijuana, causing memory loss, 75
mariposas, 220, 221, 267
marriage
  and choices, 159
  of elders, 155
  and happiness, 237
  and personal property, 160
  reasons for, 133
  reasons for leaving, 138, 236
Maslow, Abraham
  hierarchy of needs, 247, 267
  process of self-actualization, theorized, 199, 247–248
massages, 99, 114, 143, 144–146, 263
Match.com, dating service, 137
Maugham, William Somerset, 50
Mayer, Kate, viii

MayoClinic.com, 119
MCI (mild cognitive impairment), 90–91
  causing memory loss, 76
  definition of, 268
meaning, finding, 6, 46, 250
Mearns, Hughes, 55
Medicaid, 195, 203, 267
medical benefits, of caregiver, 71
Medicare, 195–196, 203, 207, 267
medications
  and aging, 99
  causing memory loss, 75
  delivering, 104
  for dementia, 53, 164
  for erectile dysfunction, 97, 134–135, 262, 273
  illicit use of, 83, 111, 204, 268
  interaction of, 44–45, 261
  L-Dopa, 98
  precautions using, 110
meditation, 84, 108, 112–114, 172, 190–191, 267
The Meeting (poem) (Shapira), 63
Mel (case study), depression, 43–44
melanoma, 94, 267
Memantine HCL (Namenda), drug, 53, 269
memory
  definition of, 267
  improving, 101–104
memory book, 77, 102
memory loss
  with aging, 73–75, *74ill*
  caregivers for person with, 68–71
  causes of, 52, 75–77
  changes due to, 66–67
  cognitive testing for, 59
  disease warning signs, 91–92
  evaluation and treatment of, 61–66
  genetic testing for, 58–59
  impact of, 51–52, 56–57
  therapy, 53–54
  things to do about, 77
  types of, 61

mental disorders, 56, 270, 271
mental health, 41–42, 107, 110, 215, 267
mental stimulation, 65, 102
meridians (energy channels), 115, 257, 267
mescal, 190
methyltrexate, 97, 267
Mexico, Days of the Dead celebration, 189–190, 261
micromanage, 40, 267
migraines, 117, 200, 268
mild cognitive impairment (MCI), 76, 90–91, 268
Miller, Henry, 147
mission statement, family, 171
MMPI (Minnesota Multi-Phasic Inventory), 72, 268
Mnemonics, 101
moles, 93–94
money, 81, 149, 194, 195, 217, 222, 234
morphine, 111, 204, 268
Morris (Uncle) "Uncle Pep," 25–26, *34ph*
MP3 players, putting thoughts on, 77
MRI (Magnetic Resonance Imaging), 53, 88, 90, 268
multiple myeloma, 93, 268
muscles, 99, 110, 117, 120, 220–221, 244, 268

N

Namenda (Memantine HCL), drug, 53
  See also NMDA-Receptor Antagonist
names
  forgetting, 74, 77
  remembering, 90
Nani, definition of, 268
  See also Wilks, Evelyn
napping, 102
neck, 1, 3, 116–117
Neruda, Pablo
  Yellow Heart, The, 100–101

nervous system, autonomic, 260, 265, 268
neurologists, 45, 59, 268
neuro-research, amygdala, 75
New York Post, 228
Newton, Sir Isaac, 37
Nintendo games, 102
Nirvana, 47
NMDA-Receptor Antagonist (N-methyl D-aspartate), 53, 269
noble truths, 47
notes, making, 102
nurturing, 67, 143, 160, 247–249
nutrition *See* diets

O

O Fortitude (poem) (Shapira), 85
Oaxaca, Mexico. Days of the Dead celebration, 189–190, 261
Obama, President, 83
obesity, 228
objectives, 156, 169, 171, 174–175
octogenarians, 50, 269
omega-3, 91
On Love (poem) (Shapira), 158–159
Oranges Are Not The Only Fruit (Winterson), 227
organize, 102
organs, 115, 125, 162, 265, 266, 270, 272
osteoarthritis, 97
Our Universe (poem) (Shapira), 192
overweight, 125, 137
  See also diets
Oxford American Desk Dictionary and Thesaurus, The, definition of
  benevolence, 16
  brain, 51
  death, 182
  dignity, 238

P

pain
  and acupuncture, 114–117, 257
  and chiropractic care, 117
  emotional, 181, 185–187, 190, 198, 200–201, 206–207
  and hypnosis, 114
  and laughter, 20
  medications, 75, 97–98
  and meditation, 113
  and migraines, 117, 200, 268
  relief of, 202, 224
  sciatica, 271
pain-free disease, 95–96
pancreas, 123, 261
paradigms, aging, 7, *9ill*
paranoid delusions, 56
Parkinson's disease, 98–99, 108, 124, 203, 263, 269
Passages (Sheehy), 6
patience, 26, 48, 67, 101, 197
pediatricians, 269
pedometer, 121, 127
pedometers, 121, 127
peer counselors, 55, 56, 269
penis, 133, 134, 135, 262, 273
perceptions
  about family members, 170, 172
  different, 64
  and fear of unknown, 181
  of normal, 51, 199
  person's, 172
  as reality, 224, 245, 250
  and Schizophrenia, 271
  of the world, 32, 41, 42
periodontal disease, 82–83, 95–96
peritoneal cavity, 203–204, 270
peritonitis, 203–204
Perlman, Itzhak, 108
personal
  experiences, 81, 88, 219, 245
  history, 38, 253
  hygiene, of caregiver, 72
  property, 159–160, 273
  references,, of caregiver, 72
  skills, of caregiver, 72
  space, 235
  strength, 95
  trainer, 127

values, 95
personality
  changes, 88, 91
  testing, 72
  traits, 268
pestilence, 79, 269
phoenix, 198, 269
physicians, 269
physiology, 52, 92, 111, 117, 238, 269
Pilates, 102
Pittsburgh, Jewish Home for the Aged, 18
pituitary gland, 51, 269
planning, 139, 174–175, 177–179, 241
plastic surgery, 80, 94, 234, 244
PMS (premenstrual syndrome), 270
poems, 102
Ponce de Leon, 92
positive attitude, 101
positive self talk, 6
Post Traumatic Stress Disorder (PTSD), 76, 87, 264
power of attorney, 178, 193, 270
prefrontal cortex, 212
prehistoric, 270
prioritizing, 74, 77, 174–175
proactive, be, 110
Project Read, 225
property, protecting, 159–160, 178, 248, 273, 274
prostate cancer, 91
proteins, 53, 124, 263
protocols, 270
protoplasm, 270
psyche, 8, 13, 22, 150, 190, 199, 244, 270
psychiatrists, 45–46, 59, 153, 182, 240, 270
psychologists, 6, 41, 59, 162, 270
psychoses, 98, 270
PTSD (Post Traumatic Stress Disorder), 76, 87, 264

Q
quality
  definition of, 271
  of exercise, 120
  herbs, 216
  of life, 124
  time, 165
quantity, 271

R
RA (rheumatoid arthritis), 85, 96–98, 263, 267, 271
Ralph (Cousin), 31, *34ph*
Readers Digest, 166
reading, 102
realizations, 43, 46–47, 199
receipts, for caregiver services, 70
references, for Home Health Agencies, 73
references, personal, of caregiver, 72
regular exercise, 83, 102, 109, 120–123, 126–127
reincarnation, 217
relationships
  complacency about, 138–139, 216
  cultivating, 215–216
  five great, 175–176
  good, 141–142, 156–161
  initial, 131
  long-term, 140, 150
  nature of, 236–237
  rules of engagement, 153–154
  sexual, 131, 132, 133–134, 146–147
relax
  learn to, 102
  taking hot shower, 190
  through meditation, 113–114
  using paraffin wax, 99
Rember, drug, 53
reminders, external, 77, 101
Reminyl (Galantamine), drug, 53
resentment, 170, 188
responsibility
  for choices, 159
  and feelings, 160
  of helping others, 247
  learning to take, 170, 171, 172

retirement, 155, 210–211, 215, 218
rheumatoid arthritis (RA), 85, 96–98,
  263, 267, 271
rhymes, 101
Rivastigmine (Exelon) drug, 53
Road Not Taken (Frost), 35–36
Rogers, Will, 81
Rollo, May, 162
routines, regular, 102

S

salary, of caregiver, 70–72
Sam (case study), transcending
  perceptions, 199–200
San Francisco Dolphin Running Club,
  110
Saunders, Dame Cicely, 202
Schaar, John, 207
schizophrenia, 56, 271
Schweitzer, Albert, 105
sciatica, 271
screening caregivers, 71–73
secret of the world, 227
selenium, 91, 271
self, inner, 46, 142, 199
self-actualization, process of, 199,
  247–248
  See also Maslow, Abraham
self-awareness, 22
self-esteem, 231, 235–236, 238, 248,
  267
self-love, 110, 148, 160–161, 240,
  247–248
self-renewal, 36–37
self-sufficiency, 214, 231
senility, 261, 271
Senility Prayer, 209, 211
"senior moments," 90
sense of initiative, 41
Serenity Prayer, 219
serum, 122, 266
the seven gifts, 241–242
sex
  act, 5, 143, 145, 146
  being prepared for, 133–136

drive, 111
and intimacy, 130–133, 143–146
sexual
  dysfunctions, 97, 134–135, 262, 273
  relationships, 131, 132, 133–134,
    146–147
sexually transmitted diseases (STDs),
  97, 134, 139, 272
Shapira, Betty (Mother), vii, *11ph*,
  25ph, *34ph*
  childhood of, 20–22
  death of husband, 140, 185–187,
    205–206
  diagnosing own disease, 54
  relationships, as widow, 140–141
  in support group, 198
  in trusting relationship, 131
Shapira, Carol (Sister-in-law), vii
Shapira, Eric Zane, *11ph*, *34ph*, 128
  on adding years to life, 109
  I Am (poem), 201–202
  I Am Alone (poem), 67
  The Meeting (poem), 63
  O Fortitude (poem), 85
  On Love (poem), 158–159
  Our Universe (poem), 192
  The Silent Sufferer (poem), 67
Shapira, Griffin (Grandson), vii
Shapira, Harvey (Brother), vii, *11ph*,
  34ph
Shapira, Irving (Father), vii, *11ph*, *25ph*,
  34ph
  death of, 140, 184–187, 205–206
  family history of, 13–14, 17
  response to something wrong, 37,
    176
  surgeries of, 88
  in trusting relationship, 131
  verbalizing feelings, 148–149
Shapira, Saul "Uncle Saul," 30–31, *34ph*
Shapira, Susan (Wife), vii, 3, 93,
  131–132
Shapira, Verity (Granddaughter), vii
Shapira, Zane (Son), vii
Shapira family (author's family), *34ph*

author, *11ph*
Broudy, Joe (Uncle), *28ph*, *34ph*
Broudy, Leah (Aunt), 26–27, *28ph*, *34ph*
Bubbie (Paternal Grandmother), *11ph*, 17–18, *34ph*
Danny (Cousin), 31, *34ph*
David (Cousin), 31, *34ph*
Diane (Cousin), 29
Edie (Cousin), 31, *34ph*
Franny (Aunt), 28–31
Harry (Second Cousin) "the old man," 15–16, 23
Jo (Mother-in-law), 85–86
Morris (Uncle) "Uncle Pep," 25–26, *34ph*
Ralph (Cousin), 31, *34ph*
Shapira, Betty (*See* Shapira, Betty (Mother))
Shapira, Carol (Sister-in-law), vii
Shapira, Eric Zane (author) (*See* Shapira, Eric Zane)
Shapira, Griffin (Grandson), vii
Shapira, Harvey (Brother), *11ph*, 24, *34ph*
Shapira, Irving (*See* Shapira, Irving (Father))
Shapira, Saul "Uncle Saul," 31, *34ph*
Shapira, Susan (Wife), vii, 3, 93, 131–132
Shapira, Verity (Granddaughter), vii
Shapira, Zane (Son), vii
Wilks, Evelyn "Nani," 19–22, *19ph*, 24–25
Wilks, Jacob "Pappa," 21–22, 24–25
Zalig, Asher (Paternal Grandfather), 13–14, 16
shared love, 205, 207
Shaw, George Bernard, 147
Sheehy, Gail
Passages, 6
Shivah, 189, 272
short-term goals, 174–175, 177
short-term memory loss, 91
side effects, drug, 97, 98, 135

significant emotional experiences, 95
The Silent Sufferer (poem) (Shapira), 67
silent sufferers, 67, 185, 198
Sister "Mary What's-Her-Name" (case study), on risky change, 209–210
skills, personal, of caregiver, 72
sleep, 12, 102
SMART, steps in goal setting, 168–170
smoking, 102, 125, 126
Socrates, 55
Solana, Joan, vii
speech center, 61, 86–87
spiritual
  suffering, relief of, 202
  values, 107, 247
  Wills, 196 (*See also* Wills)
Spock, Benjamin, 188
stages of dying, theory, 182–183
stages of intimacy, 145–146
Stanford University, 114
stationary bicycling, 102
statistics
  baby boomers, 37
  changing professions, 36
  chronic illness of Americans, 125
  definition of, 272
  fastest growing population cohort, 23
  life-span, 11, 83, 96, 109, 245
  suicide rates, 233
  women being alone, 152
STDs (sexually transmitted diseases), 97, 134, 139, 272
steroids, 112, 113, 272
stimulation, mental, 65, 102, 103
strength, inner, 6, 42, 230, 246
stress
  and "boomer triangle," 244
  and cortisol, 260
  exercise reducing, 120
  in family crisis, *163ill*, 164–167, 173
  meditation reducing, 112–114
  and memory loss, 76, 102
  psychological, 45–47
  PTSD (Post Traumatic Stress Disorder), 87, 264

and self-actualization, 199
and a short life, 112
and worry, 238
stressors, 177, 179
strokes
   CVA (cerebral vascular accident), 61, 260
   and dementia, 76–77
   and durable power of healthcare, 193
   L-Dopa drugs and, 98
   and speech center of brain, 86–87
   TIAs (transient ischemic attacks), 53, 61, 75, 86, 88, 273
sucrose, 123–124
Sudoku, 102, 212, 224
suicides, 45, 188
support groups, 103, 198
Surgeon General, 272
Surgeon General, U.S., 13, 83
survivors, 40, 45–46, 188–191
Swartz, Don, 150
swimming, 102
Swindoll, Charles, 184
   Heart To Heart, 48
SWOT analysis, 174–175, 272
Sylvia (case study), respect for family, 157–158
synagogue, first in Toronto, 14
syphilis, 76, 272
systemic, 76, 82, 83, 271, 272
systemic diseases, 82, 83
   causing memory loss, 76

T

Tacrine (Cognex), drug, 53
tai chi, 102
Tau proteins, 53
Taylor-Johnson Temperament Analysis, 72
TB (tuberculosis), 76, 272
teeth, 82, 96, 97, 109, 110
Teller, Edward, 233
Ten Stages Of Intimacy, 145–146
thalamus, 74, *74ill*, 273
Thalidomide, drug, 199–200

Theory Of Relativity, 273
thirst, loss of, 51, 52
thyroid dysfunctions, causing memory loss, 76
TIAs (transient ischemic attacks), 53, 61, 75, 86, 88, 273
tissue necrosis factor, 97–98
tobacco, use of, 83
Toronto, synagogue, first in, 14
toxins, 244
trans fats, 12, 122–124
transformation, internal, 40, 41
transitions
   and changes, 40
   definition of, 273
   embracing aging, 5, 10
   in families, 167–171, 176–179
   to grieving process, 189, 198–199
   as renewal, 36, 37
Transitions (Bridges), 36
tremors, 15, 98, 99, 269
triaging patients to treat illness, 202
triglycerides, 122, 273
true happiness, 47
true love, 150–155
trust
   developing, 41, 171–172, 175
   intimacy and, 131, 133
trust, legal, 69, 178, 195, 273
truths, four noble, 47
tuberculosis (TB), 76, 272
Tuesdays with Morrie (Albom), 205
tumors, 80, 259, 265

U

United States (U.S.)
   caregivers in, 69, 73
   death celebration of life, 189
   Medicare and Medicaid benefits in, 203
   vs. Chinese medicine, 116
"universe," 228
"the unthinkable," 54
U.S. Census Bureau, 37
U.S. Surgeon General, 13, 83, 272

USO (United Service Organization), 225, 273

V
valid drivers license, of caregiver, 71–72
validate, 273
values
  after a trauma, 32
  determining relationship, 156
  discovering core family, 171, 173, 224
  habits and, 230
  spiritual, 107, 247
Van Buren, Abigail, 171
Viagra, 97, 273
victims, 76, 203, 229, 230–231, 249
Virtues of Aging, The (Carter), 251
Viscott, David, 153
vision statement, family, 171
visioning, 3, 32, 241
visualizations, 101, 112, 114, 190–191, 213, 264
vitamins, 75–76, 91, 103, 109, 127, 274
Von Foerster, Heinz, 51, 55, 181

W
walking
  benefits of, 3, 168
  as part of exercise program, 102, 120–122, 214, 224
  as part of healthy lifestyle, 86, 92, 126, 128
WebMD, 119
white blood cells, 266
Wicker, John, 217
widows, 140, 150, 157, 194
Wilks, Evelyn "Nani," 19–22, *19ph*, 24–25
Wilks, Jacob "Pappa," *19ph*, 21–22, 24–25
will, autonomous, 41
will to change, 43
Williams, Robin, 132–133
Wills, 194–196, 274

Willson, Meredith, 241–242
wine, health benefits from, 65, 119, 125
Winterson, Jeanette
  Oranges Are Not The Only Fruit, 227
wisdom
  definition of, 246, 274
  and dignity, 226
  of elders, 7, 179, 240, 262
  and experience, in sexual activity, 97
  and making a difference in life, 218–219
  as reference for others, 245
  and understanding, 32–33
worker's compensation insurance, for caregiver, 71
world, secret of the, 227
worrying, 179, 238
Wright, Frank Lloyd, 10
Wright, Steven, 219
wrinkles, 244, 274
writing poems, 102

Y
Yeats, William Butler, 130
Yellow Heart, The (Neruda), 100–101
Yiddish, 274
yin-yang, 58, 115, 274
YMCAs, 127
yoga, 102

Z
Zalig, Asher (Paternal Grandfather), 13–14, 16
zest, 36, 214–216
zymurgy, 173, 274
Zymurgy Society, 173